Pocket Picture Guides
to Clinical Medicine

Rheumatic Diseases

Pocket Picture Guides
to Clinical Medicine

Rheumatic Diseases

Michael Shipley MA, MD, MRCP

Consultant Rheumatologist,
The Middlesex Hospital, London, UK

Gower Medical Publishing · London · New York · 1984

ISBN 0-906923-15-8

British Library Cataloguing in Publication Data
Shipley, Michael
    Rheumatic diseases. –
    (Pocket Picture Guides to Clinical Medicine; 2)
    I. Title   II. Series
    616.7'23   RC 927

Project Editor: Fiona Carr
    Designer: Teresa Foster
    Illustrator: Jeremy Cort

Originated in Hong Kong by Imago Publishing Ltd.
Printed in Great Britain by W. S. Cowell Ltd.

Pocket Picture Guides
to Clinical Medicine

The purpose of this series is to provide essential visual information about commonly encountered diseases in a convenient practical and economic format. Each Pocket Picture Guide covers an important area of day-to-day clinical medicine. The main feature of these books is the superbly photographed colour reproductions of typical clinical appearances. Other visual diagnostic information, such as X-rays, is included where appropriate. Each illustration is fully explained by a clearly written descriptive caption highlighting important diagnostic features. Tables presenting other diagnostic and differential diagnostic information are included where appropriate. A comprehensive and carefully compiled index makes each Pocket Picture Guide an easy to use source of visual reference.

An extensive series is planned and other titles in the initial group of Pocket Picture Guides are:

Infectious Diseases
Sexually Transmitted Diseases
Skin Diseases
Paediatrics

Acknowledgements

The author would like to thank the following colleagues for providing illustrative material: Prof. A. W. Asscher, K.R.U.F. Institute, Royal Infirmary, Cardiff (Fig. 5.6); Prof. P. A. Bacon, Department of Rheumatology, The University of Birmingham, Birmingham (Fig. 2.33); Dr. A. N. Bamji, Department of Rheumatology and Rehabilitation, The Brook General Hospital, London (Fig. 3.17 right); Dr. A. C. Boyle, Department of Rheumatology, The Middlesex Hospital, London (Fig. 2.1), Mr. J. P. Browett, Orthopaedic Department, St. Bartholomew's Hospital, London (Fig. 2.10), Dr. P. A. Dieppe, Department of Rheumatology, Bristol Royal Infirmary, Bristol (Figs. 1.1, 1.8, 1.11, 1.12, 2.13, 2.20, 2.24, 2.32, 5.1, 5.2, 5.5, 5.7); Prof. M. I. V. Jayson, Rheumatic Diseases Centre, University of Manchester, Salford (Figs. 4.20, 4.26); Dr. J. T. Scott, Kennedy Institute of Rheumatology, London (Fig. 5.2 right); Dr. I. Watt, Department of Radiodiagnosis Bristol Royal Infirmary, Bristol (1.3, 1.5, 1.13, 2.6, 4.13, 4.14).

Contents

Introduction

A rheumatologist sees a wide variety of diseases and complaints; their diagnosis and management is a constant challenge. Although frequently self-limiting and rarely fatal, the rheumatic diseases are common and cause considerable pain and suffering. They can, however, be alleviated by early diagnosis and prompt intervention.

Pain is a symptom common to most of these complaints and often anxiety and depression about possible progressive disability must be recognised, and reassurance given whenever possible. Indeed, some cases will require little more than reassurance and simple physical measures such as support, rest, heat or various physiotherapeutic techniques. At the other end of the spectrum the diagnosis of, for example, rheumatoid arthritis, may mark the beginning of a lifetime's relationship between the patient and his or her medical advisers. Reassurance in such cases must be tempered with realism, although fortunately the rapidly progressive case leading to severe disability is rare and many such patients lead relatively normal lives. RA is still incurable in 1983, but the patient should certainly not be left without hope.

Drugs are playing an increasingly important part in the management of painful inflammatory conditions but of late, their relative lack of efficacy in some cases, and potential for producing side-effects in others, are leading to disillusionment amongst patients. Analgesic and anti-inflammatory agents are undoubtedly valuable therapeutic tools. However, their excessive and inappropriate use may eventually bring them into disrepute and thus limit the freedom of the medical profession to prescribe them for the more severe inflammatory disorders, where they do definitely bring comfort and relief.

It is hoped that the pictorial format of this handbook will provide clues on how to approach the management of some of the commoner rheumatic problems and suggest when specialist referral might be advisable. Clinical pictures have been supplemented where appropriate with diagrams or tables to provide convenient visual reference and aides memoires.

Osteoarthritis of peripheral synovial joints

Osteoarthritis produces a wide variety of symptoms; these are often mild, and may require little more than reassurance from the doctor, but symptomatic OA is common with increasing age and is a significant cause of pain and misery in the elderly. It causes the loss of several million working days every year and is the most common cause of disability in the United Kingdom. Genetic factors appear to be involved in the aetiology but they are complex, and there is a wide geographic variation of both joint distribution and prevalence. The prevalence is particularly high in the UK. Trauma due to fracture through the joint or caused by certain sporting activities, congenital abnormalities or joint damage from pre-existing infective or inflammatory arthritis may predispose a patient to the development of OA.

OA of peripheral synovial joints develops after an initially reversible phase during which fibrillation of the articular cartilage occurs. This change is associated with specific biochemical and histological abnormalities of the cartilage. Subsequent destruction of the articular cartilage leads to sclerosis and remodelling of the exposed sub-chondral bone. Periarticular osteophyte formation and a variable degree of synovial inflammation also occur. Recent work has suggested that an inflammatory component may be involved in the development of this disease and that crystals of calcium hydroxyapatite may either initiate or perpetuate the inflammation. Biochemical studies are also beginning to shed some light on this process and prevention may eventually become feasible. In the meantime, treatment is by analgesic and non-steroidal anti-inflammatory agents, the use of which should be continually reviewed to see whether their prescription is indeed still beneficial. Physiotherapy has a role to play but is usually only helpful for a brief period after completion of the treatment. Surgery offers the greatest hope in the patient whose pain or disability is sufficient to warrant it, but the greatest challenge lies in the management of those patients whose pain both on movement and at night is a cause of persistent distress, but in whom surgery is not yet indicated.

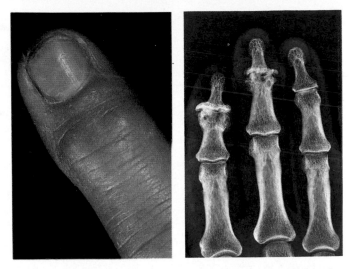

Fig. 1.1 Heberden's nodes are the commonest manifestation of osteoarthritis presenting to a doctor. They occur mainly in women over the age of 50. Initially painful, they usually result in painless stiffening and occasionally instability. Typical radiological changes are loss of joint space, sclerosis, osteophytes and cystic changes.

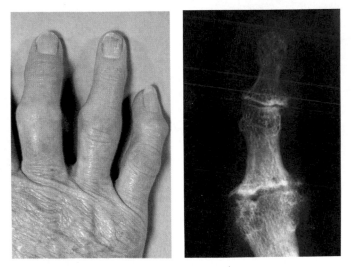

Fig. 1.2 Less commonly, the proximal interphalangeal (PIP) joints are involved with bony swelling (Bouchard's nodes) and have similar radiological appearances. Such involvement is often a cause of concern to the patient who fears a more generalised disease and resultant disability. Fortunately this is relatively uncommon and reassurance is usually possible.

2

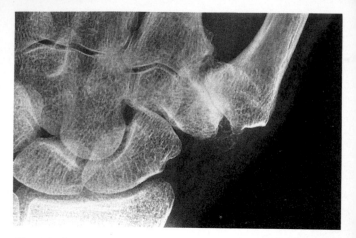

Fig. 1.3 Osteoarthritis of the first carpometacarpal (CMC) joint, again more common in women, frequently causes pain at the base of the thumb. Local steroid injection may help but usually the joint becomes stiff with the thumb adducted, giving the hand a typically square appearance. Occasionally surgery is indicated in severe cases.

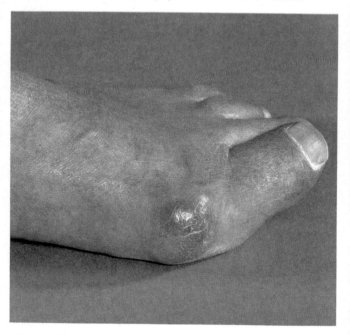

Fig. 1.4 OA of the first metatarsophalangeal (MTP) joints leads to either hallux rigidus or to a hallux valgus deformity when the overlying painful bursa (bunion) may be a source of discomfort.

3

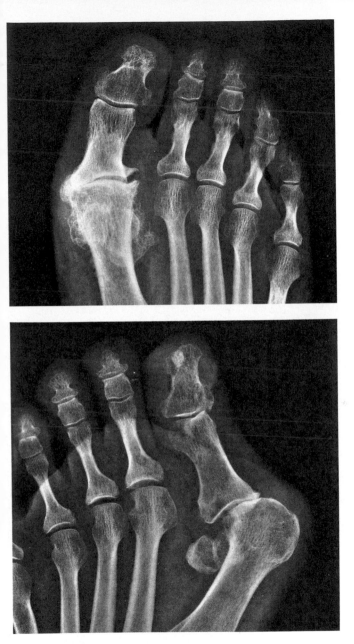

Fig. 1.5 Hallux rigidus is often associated with a degree of valgus deformity but the radiological appearance with florid osteophyte formation (upper) distinguishes it from simple hallux valgus (lower).

4

Factors predisposing to osteoarthritis	
Trauma	Fracture through joint Meniscus injury / surgery Joint instability Occupational and sporting
Congenital anomaly	Congenital hip dislocation Epiphyseal dysplasia
Inflammatory arthritis	Rheumatoid arthritis
Metabolic diseases	Gout Chondrocalcinosis Acromegaly Ochronosis

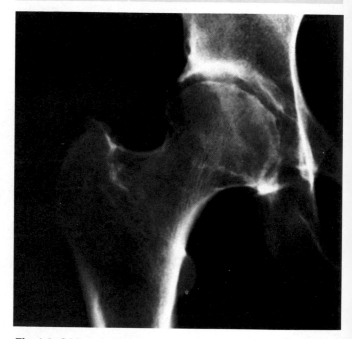

Fig. 1.6 OA is probably best thought of as the final common pathway of a variety of predisposing factors which lead, via cartilage damage, to reactive bony changes. Its pathogenesis is multifactorial although certain predisposing factors can be identified. Here, acromegaly is associated with irregularity of the bone surfaces despite normal cartilage thickness.

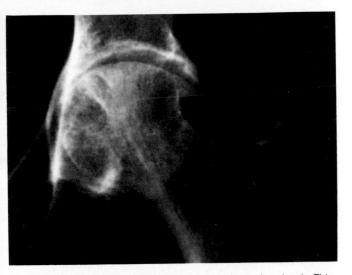

Fig. 1.7 OA of the hip initially causes pain in the buttock and groin. This pain may radiate to the knee, which is occasionally the main site of referred pain, causing confusion and delay in diagnosis. Radiologically there is loss of joint space which may be concentric, superior or occasionally central as shown here.

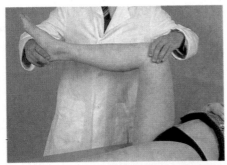

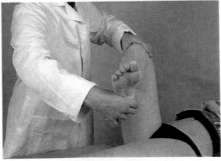

Fig. 1.8 Clinical examination early in the disease may be unremarkable, but reduced internal and external rotation can often be detected with the hip flexed. The procedure may reproduce the patient's pain, which is present mainly on weight-bearing at this stage.

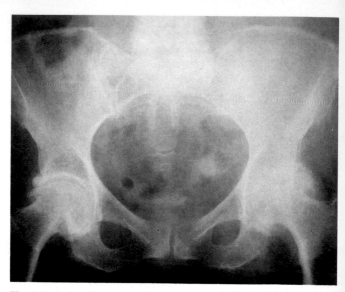

Fig. 1.9 As the disease advances further, so florid osteophyte formation may limit movement of the joint. The patient finds it difficult to reach his foot to tie shoe laces, put on socks or stockings etc. Night pain may become troublesome.

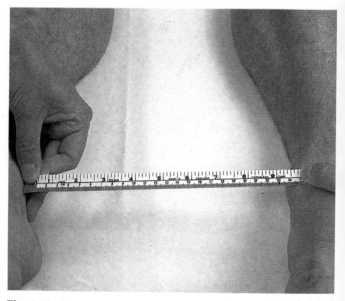

Fig. 1.10 Gross limitation of abduction can be measured directly as the intermalleolar distance. More rarely, fixed abduction occurs.

7

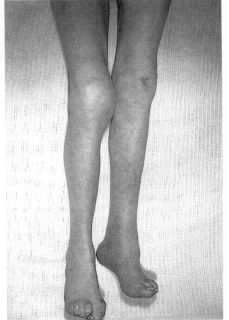

Fig. 1.11 There is often fixed adduction, flexion and external rotation which leads to pelvic tilting and apparent shortening of the affected leg. Back pain often results and there may be stressing of the opposite knee leading to further pain and disability (the so-called 'long leg' syndrome).

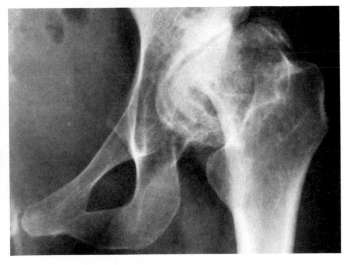

Fig. 1.12 Premature OA of the hip is often associated with some predisposing factor; here a patient with previously undiagnosed congenital dislocation of the hip (CDH) demonstrates resultant deformity of the femoral head and OA. Such cases make the early detection and management of CDH essential.

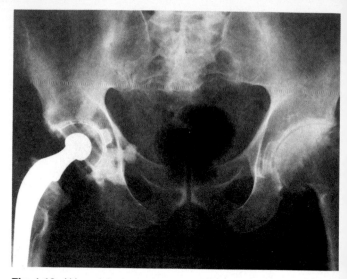

Fig. 1.13 Although in some younger patients a femoral osteotomy may produce a few years of relief, total hip replacement (THR) is the best course for most when pain and disability are intolerable. The patient has received a right Charnley prosthesis.

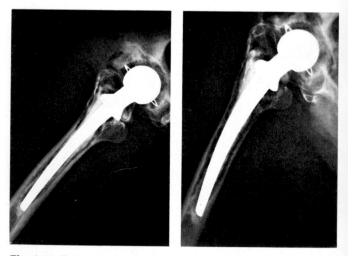

Fig. 1.14 The long-term results of THR are now very satisfactory with only 10-15% failure at 10 years due to loosening and/or infection. Reoperation is often feasible but these risks still mean that THR in an active younger patient must be very carefully weighed up and discussed. The X-rays show the hip of a 35 year old woman who received a THR five years prior to the left X-ray. Two years later (right) the widened lucent zone reflects loosening.

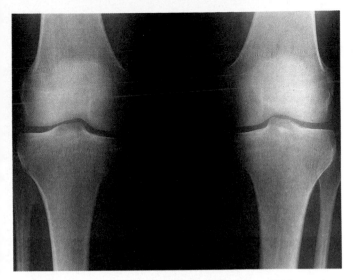

Fig. 1.15 Knee X-rays with the patient standing are useful for demonstrating cartilage thickness and weight-bearing deformity. In these normal knees, there is no reduction of medial and lateral cartilage thickness, the tibial spines are smooth and alignment is normal.

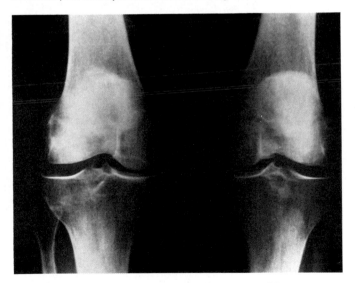

Fig. 1.16 By contrast, this patient demonstrates two of the common early features of OA: spiking of the tibial spines and loss of thickness of the medial articular cartilage, which leads on to a varus deformity. In selected early cases tibial osteotomy redistributes the weight and may delay progression.

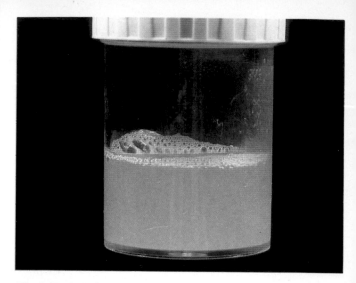

Fig. 1.17 At times a more inflammatory picture supervenes with the development of a joint effusion. Usually this is clear and viscous (unlike the cloudy, thin effusion of RA). A very hot knee may be due to a haemarthrosis or to coincident pseudogout. Diagnostic aspiration is necessary and corticosteroid injection may be indicated (see Fig. 5.12).

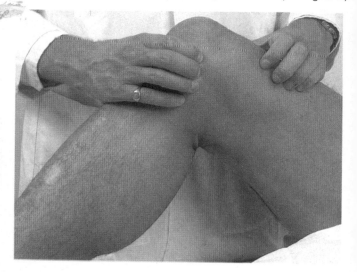

Fig. 1.18 The pain of an osteoarthritic knee may arise from the tibio-femoral and/or patello femoral articulations but is often also due to soft tissue problems. Pain at the insertion of the collateral ligaments is common and areas of local tenderness may be helped by locally injected lignocaine and corticosteroid.

11

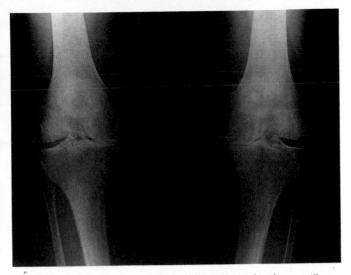

Fig. 1.19 With more advanced disease, total loss of surface cartilage with subchondral eburnation develops. This bone is less resilient and is likely to fracture under stress, increasing the tendency towards varus deformity and weight-bearing through the already stressed medial tibial plateau.

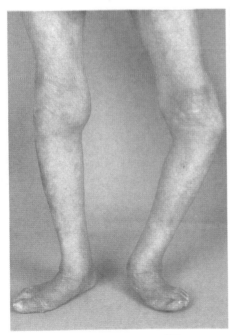

Fig. 1.20 This typical varus deformity with bony swelling in long-standing OA is painful, unstable and thus very disabling. Total knee replacement despite its risks is the only procedure which will help but the patient must be warned not to stress the prosthesis unduly.

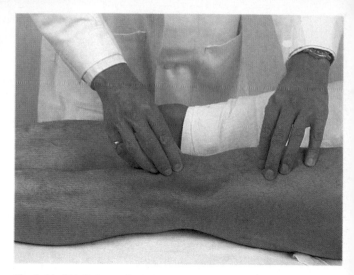

Fig. 1.21 Patellofemoral pain is often troublesome on stairs and when getting up from a chair. It can be elicited by direct pressure over the patella, with the patient actively contracting the quadriceps. In young adults this is often due to chondromalacia patellae which is usually self-limiting.

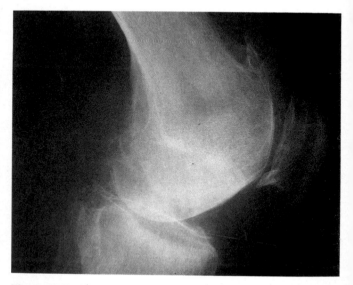

Fig. 1.22 Florid osteophyte formation may occasionally be seen and is often a feature of generalised osteoarthritis (GOA). There is uncertainty about factors which predispose to isolated patellofemoral OA—the role of previous chondromalacia is probably slight.

13

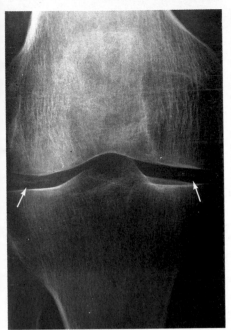

Fig. 1.23 OA of the knees may be seen in sportsmen, especially footballers, in women who have primary generalised osteoarthritis, (which tends to run in families and of which Heberden's nodes are a diagnostic marker), or, as here, in a patient with chondrocalcinosis secondary to hyperparathyroidism.

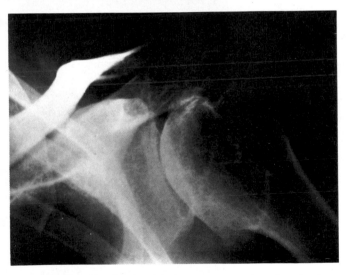

Fig. 1.24 OA of the shoulder joint is uncommon unless there has been predisposing trauma. This patient fractured the humerus but did not seek advice for two years when she presented with an immobile shoulder. Radiological changes show deformity of the head of the humerus and osteophyte formation.

14

Rheumatoid arthritis

Rheumatoid arthritis occurs more commonly in women than in men. Although it may present at any age, it is rare in prepubertal children and usually occurs in women during the childbearing years. The typically symmetrical and peripheral polyarthritis is often associated with marked morning stiffness, malaise and a normochromic, normocytic anaemia. At initial presentation, the symptoms have usually been present for several months but still may not be diagnostic. The pattern of progression of the disease is important in distinguishing it from the self-limiting polyarthritis which may follow such viral illnesses as rubella, and from the chronic, but usually less disabling, arthritis of this peripheral and symmetrical type, which may be associated with psoriasis. The type of therapy used depends upon the type of arthritis, hence it is important to observe the changes seen over the early months before committing the patient to the more toxic drugs which are usually necessary in treating rheumatoid arthritis.

Although the commonest of the inflammatory polyarthritides, it is unlikely that more than one new case of thisunpredictable, sometimes disabling disease will present to the average general practitioner per year. In consequence, his experience of its management and of the manipulation of drug treatment is inevitably limited. These patients need the support which the GP can give them locally but they also need the additional care of a specialist who, because of his larger pool of patients, is better placed to recognise poor prognostic signs and complications, and advise on their management. The aim of the following section is to give pointers to the early recognition of rheumatoid arthritis and also to emphasise those clinical features requiring specialist attention and those which can be helped by surgery and other means.

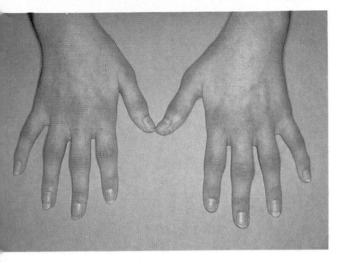

Fig. 2.1 Swelling of the metacarpophalangeal (MCP) joints and the proximal interphalangeal (PIP) joints, leading to filling in of the hollows between the knuckles and 'spindling' of the fingers is typical, but not diagnostic, of early rheumatoid arthritis. The feet, wrists, knees, elbows and shoulders may also become involved. Morning stiffness is a distressing associated symptom.

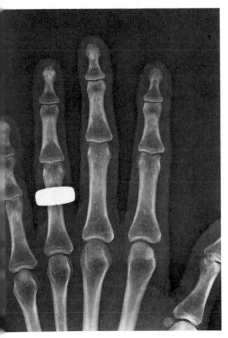

Fig. 2.2 Radiological changes in the early stages are usually limited to soft tissue swelling and juxta-articular osteoporosis. These changes are typical of, but not specific to, early rheumatoid arthritis.

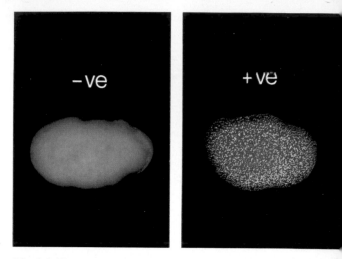

Fig. 2.3 The presence of IgM anti-globulins (rheumatoid factors) in the serum of patients with symmetrical polyarthritis usually but not always implies that they have rheumatoid arthritis. The test involves the agglutination of either sheep red cells coated in rabbit anti-sheep antibody (SCAT) or as here, of latex particles coated with human IgG. IgG and IgA rheumatoid factors are also found but are more difficult to detect. They may provide useful prognostic and diagnostic information in the future.

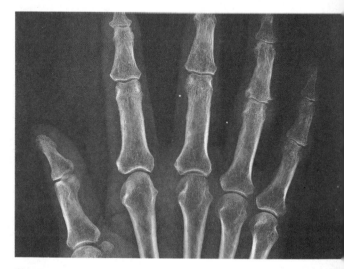

Fig. 2.4 Erosions, one of the hallmarks of rheumatoid arthritis, may not appear for 6-12 months, or even longer in the milder case. They should be looked for in the hands, wrists and feet. Here, early erosions are seen around the PIP joints of the ring and little fingers.

17

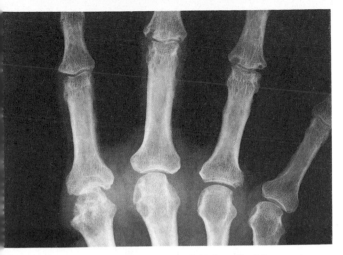

Fig. 2.5 Typically, bone erosions occur initially at the joint margins where the capsule is attached. Later the inflamed synovium extends across the surface of the articular cartilage (pannus formation). This first destroys the cartilage and later the underlying bone.

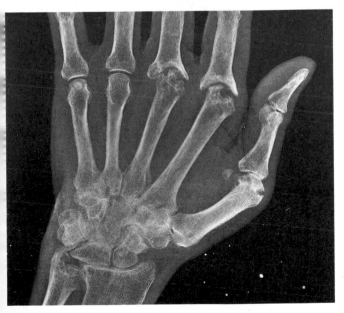

Fig. 2.6 Rheumatoid arthritis two years after the onset of the disease. There is extensive erosion of the MCP joints in the index and middle fingers. The joint space at the wrist is narrowed and there are early changes in the carpus.

18

American Rheumatism Association Criteria

Morning stiffness

Pain on motion or tenderness in at least one joint

Swelling (soft tissue thickening of fluid) in at least one joint

Swelling (observed by a physician) of at least one other joint within three months

Symmetrical joint swelling (not terminal interphalangeal joints)

Subcutaneous nodules

X-ray changes typical of rheumatoid arthritis which must include at least bony decalcification around the involved joints

Positive agglutination test – demonstration of IgM 'rheumatoid factor'

Fig. 2.7 The American Rheumatism Association criteria for the diagnosis of rheumatoid arthritis have been useful for defining cases entered into clinical trials, but are of limited value early in the disease. Cases are classified according to the number of criteria satisfied, into 'Classical' – 7, 'Definite' – 5 and 'Probable' – 3. There are 21 exclusion criteria used to avoid confusion with other causes of polyarthritis.

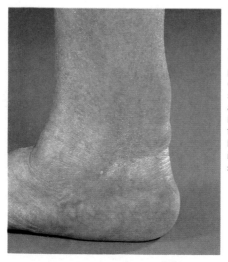

Fig. 2.8 Nodules are one of the diagnostic criteria of rheumatoid arthritis. They are usually found over pressure points, most commonly on the ulnar surface of the forearm and elbow, but also, as here, over the Achilles tendon. They are often lobulated, usually firm in consistency and subcutaneous.

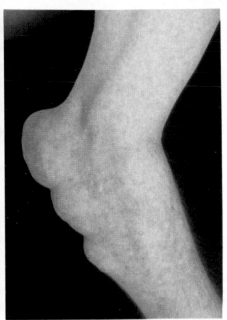

Fig. 2.9 Giant nodules are cosmetically unacceptable and tender because of repeated pressure. The overlying skin may ulcerate. Although liable to recur, they are best removed surgically.

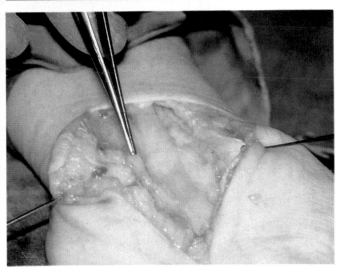

Fig. 2.10 Carpal involvement is often associated with the development of carpal tunnel syndrome due to compression of the median nerve by inflamed synovium (being held by forceps). The symptoms and method of injection for CTS are shown in Fig. 3.17. Occasionally in persistent cases where conduction studies show that motor and sensory nerve damage is severe surgical decompression is necessary.

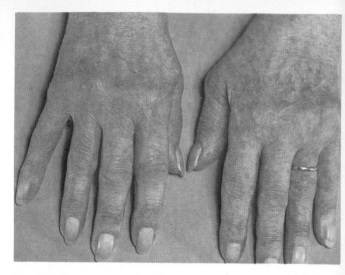

Fig. 2.11 The nature of rheumatoid arthritis in its progressive form is exemplified by the damage it can do to the hands. Here, in addition to MCP and PIP joint swelling, the little finger of the right hand is beginning to go into ulnar deviation and there is marked wasting of the small muscles of the hand.

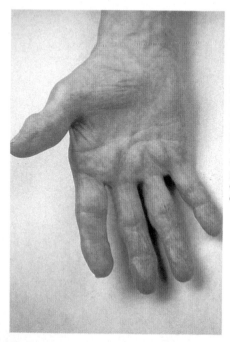

Fig. 2.12 The range of movement of the fingers becomes limited not only because of joint involvement but also because of synovitis of tendon sheaths, seen here in the finger flexors. The early local injection of corticosteroids by an expert may help to prevent or delay the development of deformity.

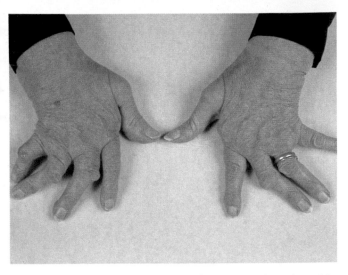

Fig. 2.13 Uncontrolled rheumatoid arthritis in the hands produces this diagnostic picture: the MCP joints have subluxed, with the digits moving towards the palm, and there is marked ulnar drift. Joint damage is apparent in the finger PIP joints and in the thumbs, which show 'Z' deformities.

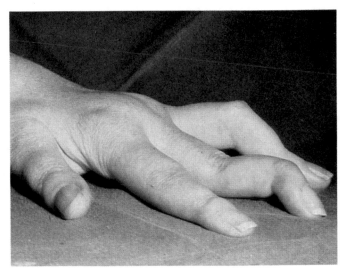

Fig. 2.14 Two of the classically described finger deformities most common in rheumatoid arthritis. The ring finger shows a boutonnière deformity with fixed flexion at the PIP joint. The middle finger shows a swan neck deformity with fixed hyperextension at the PIP and fixed flexion at the distal interphalangeal (DIP) joint.

22

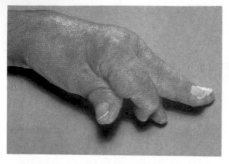

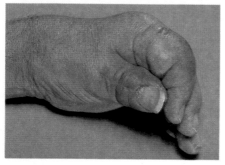

Fig. 2.15 Hand surgery by a specialised orthopaedic or plastic surgeon may improve function in selected cases and referral to a hand clinic may be considered. This patient with destructive RA has had his pinch grip restored by pinning of the IP joints of the thumb. Prevention by disease control, local injections and surgery remains the goal but is still distressingly difficult to achieve.

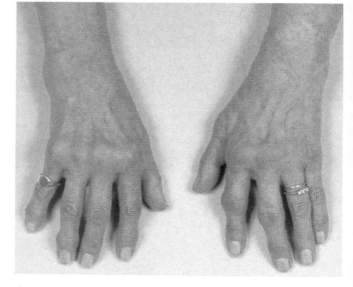

Fig. 2.16 Synovitis of the wrist is frequently seen in early rheumatoid arthritis. In addition to swelling, there is often tenderness over the ulnar styloid, which may be unstable.

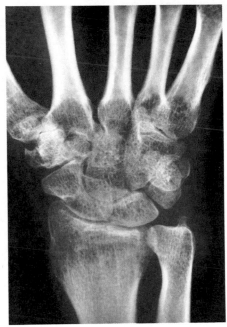

Fig. 2.17 Erosions of the ulnar styloid are often seen early in RA. When present they establish the diagnosis.

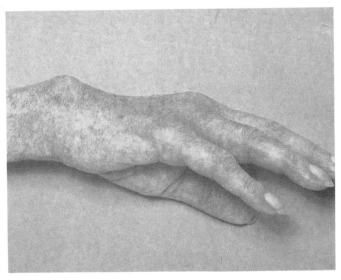

Fig. 2.18 As the inflammatory process extends from the wrist joint to involve the carpus, wrist movements become weak, painful and restricted. Subluxation of the carpus on the wrist is seen here, a deformity which impairs wrist and finger function.

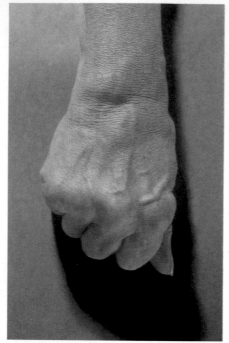

Fig. 2.19 Involvement of the extensor tendon sheaths by the rheumatoid process produces this typical hour-glass swelling: in combination with erosion of the ulnar styloid it may lead to rupture of finger extensor tendons with resultant finger drop.

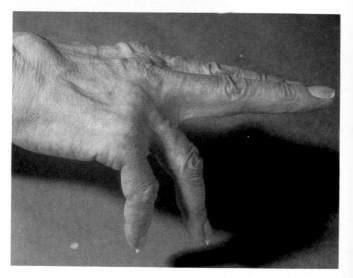

Fig. 2.20 Extensor tendon rupture. The little and ring fingers are more commonly affected. Early surgical referral is essential if satisfactory repair is to be achieved.

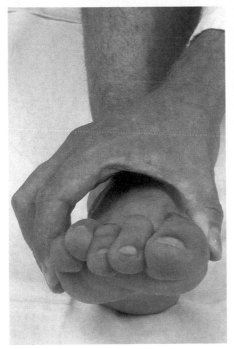

Fig. 2.21 Metatarsal pain is not limited to RA but is a common feature of it. The foot becomes broadened and there is often palpable synovial swelling. Squeezing the forefoot may elicit pain.

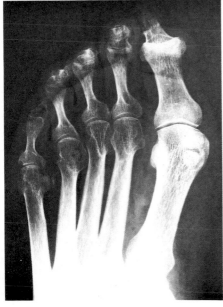

Fig. 2.22 In early rheumatoid arthritis, the metatarsal heads are occasionally the first site of erosive change to appear on X-rays. Note splaying of the metatarsal bones due to soft tissue swelling.

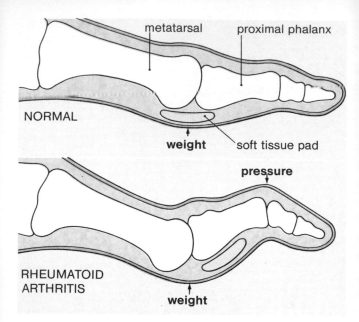

NORMAL

weight ← soft tissue pad

pressure

RHEUMATOID ARTHRITIS

weight

Fig. 2.23 Dorsal subluxation of the toes deprives the metatarsal heads of their soft tissue cushions. The bones become directly weight-bearing and the toes hammered.

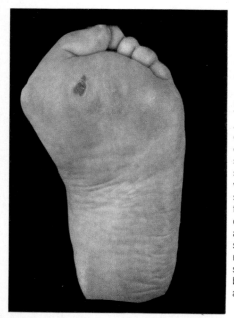

Fig. 2.24 Painful callosities develop over the subluxed metatarsal heads and the patient complains of 'walking on pebbles'. Typically, pronounced hallux valgus also develops. At this stage the discomfort may be eased by metatarsal supports or shoes with specially moulded, weight-distributing soles. Ulceration of the metatarsal callosities is often associated with severe pain and a high risk of infection. This should be avoidable by the use of appropriate surgery.

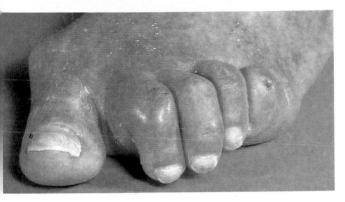

Fig. 2.25 Ulceration over the PIP joints of the hammer toes and/or over the bunion is usually caused by poor fitting shoes and adds to the misery. Shoes with soft uppers or 'space' shoes may be helpful.

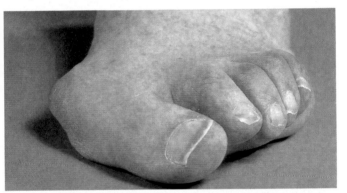

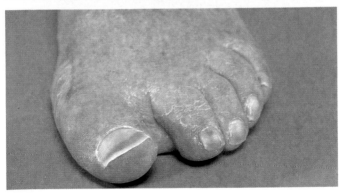

Fig. 2.26 Excision arthroplasty is an excellent operation when done well, relieving pain and often restoring normal mobility. The foot is rendered one shoe size smaller.

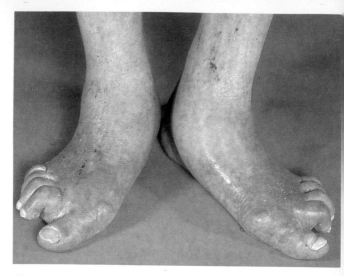

Fig. 2.27 Mid tarsal, subtaloid and ankle involvement in RA may combine to produce disabling deformity of the type seen in this patient with total collapse of the mid foot and a valgus deformity of the hind foot. With such advanced disease, modification of the footwear is the only procedure likely to benefit the patient.

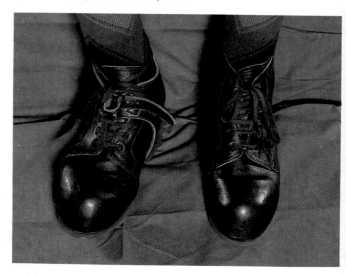

Fig. 2.28 Various types of shoe or boot are available and should be carefully selected to provide adequate space, protection and support. Here, in addition to accommodating severely deformed forefeet, T-straps have been incorporated into the boots to try and reduce the valgus deformity of the hindfoot.

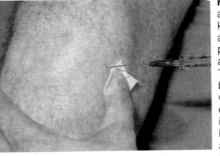

Fig. 2.29 The knee is the commonest large joint to be involved in RA. Boggy synovitis is often accompanied by an effusion which in this case is distending the suprapatellar pouch. Intra-articular corticosteroids will usually produce dramatic relief although this is usually temporary. Too frequent injection is best avoided.

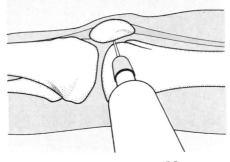

Fig. 2.30 Aspiration and injection of the knee joint are best achieved with the patient semi-reclining and the joint extended. The quadriceps must be relaxed, especially when there is no effusion, if the needle is to be introduced between the patella and the femur at the midpoint of the patella. The needle is best advanced cautiously from the medial side and inclined slightly posterolaterally as shown. The leg should be slightly externally rotated.

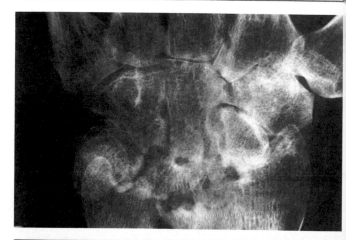

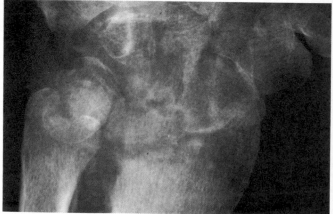

Fig. 2.31 Injection into an infected joint can lead to a sudden and rapid increase in bone damage as is seen in the wrist of this patient. The X-rays are separated by only three weeks. *Staphylococcus aureus* was grown from the exudate.

31

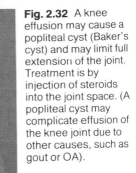

Fig. 2.32 A knee effusion may cause a popliteal cyst (Baker's cyst) and may limit full extension of the joint. Treatment is by injection of steroids into the joint space. (A popliteal cyst may complicate effusion of the knee joint due to other causes, such as gout or OA).

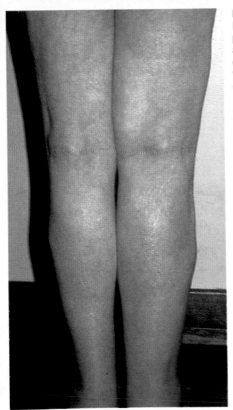

Fig. 2.33 Rupture of a Baker's cyst may produce severe pain and swelling in the calf, often associated with marked ankle oedema. This may mimic the clinical appearance of a deep venous thrombosis (DVT). Once rupture has occurred the knee effusion may disappear but the history of previous swelling of the knee and sudden onset of pain in the calf are suggestive.

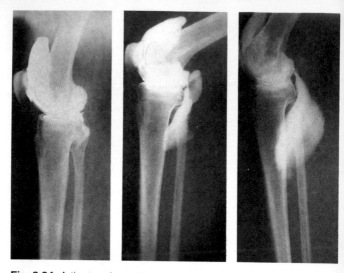

Fig. 2.34 Arthrography or ultrasonography will distinguish a ruptured cyst from a DVT – an important clinical distinction, as inappropriate treatment with heparin may lead to exacerbation of the symptoms of a ruptured cyst. This X-ray clearly shows contrast medium, which has been injected into the joint, leaking into the calf.

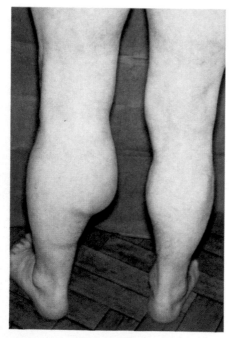

Fig. 2.35 Occasionally the cyst ruptures and slowly leaks fluid, leading to the formation of a chronic calf cyst. This is usually dealt with by surgical excision.

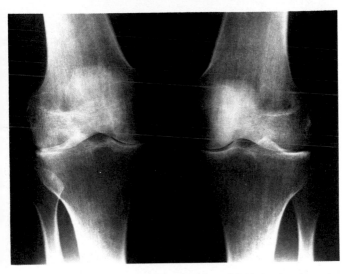

Fig. 2.36 Radiological examination of the knee joint is best performed with the patient standing – it gives a clearer picture of cartilage loss, seen here in a patient with rapidly progressive RA. Erosive changes appear late in the knees. Standing X-rays also demonstrate any deformity on weight-bearing.

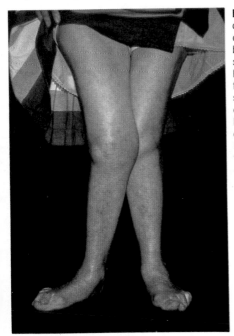

Fig. 2.37 The range of collateral instability can be assessed by medial and lateral stressing of the lower leg with the femur fixed. The patient should also always be examined standing. Here, bilateral valgus deformities of the knee are combined with valgus deformities of both hind feet. Other joint problems and the overall needs of the patient must be considered in planning the management of individual joints.

34

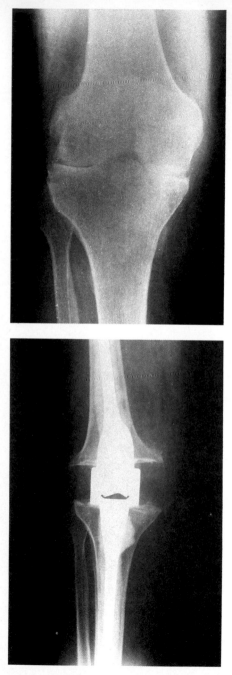

Fig. 2.38a. Synovectomy may temporarily delay progress of local disease early in its course. Once cartilage wear, erosions and deformity have developed, as here with collapse of the medial tibial plateau, surgical replacement is the procedure of choice. In selected cases this results in reduction of pain and an often dramatic improvement of mobility.

Fig. 2.38b. Here a Stanmore hinge prosthesis has been used in a relatively immobile patient.

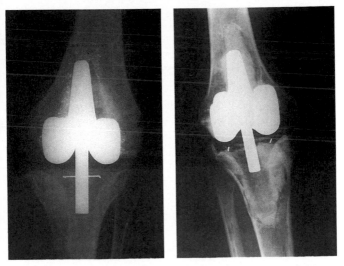

Fig. 2.39 The long-term outcome of total knee replacement (TKR) remains uncertain and such problems as fracture (left) or infection may necessitate re-replacement, arthrodesis or, rarely, amputation. Infection (right) is often preceded by the development of a lucent line around the prosthesis; or evidence of periosteal new bone formation.

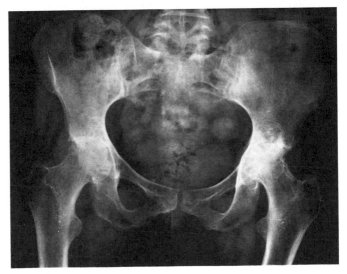

Fig. 2.40 The hip may be involved in RA with resultant pain and limitation of movement. Radiologically, there is little reactive sclerosis and symmetrical loss of the articular cartilage (compare Fig. 1.9). In advanced RA, protrusion through the pelvis may develop, making surgery technically much more difficult.

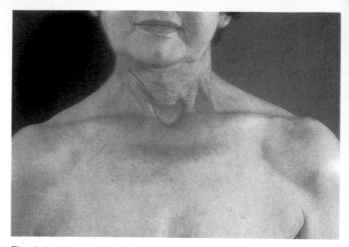

Fig. 2.41 RA of the shoulder may produce symptoms ranging from mild morning stiffness to severe pain and restriction. This patient has a large effusion in her left shoulder requiring aspiration and local injection of steroid. More commonly swelling is less marked than in this case, but pain may be severe and intra-articular injection still warranted.

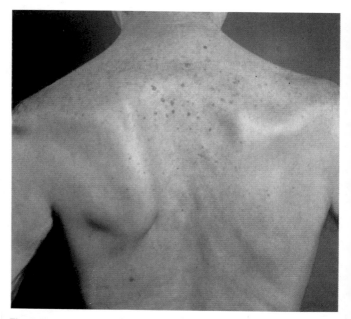

Fig. 2.42 Long-standing RA may lead to gross damage which restricts movement and is often associated with wasting of the shoulder girdle muscles, as in this patient.

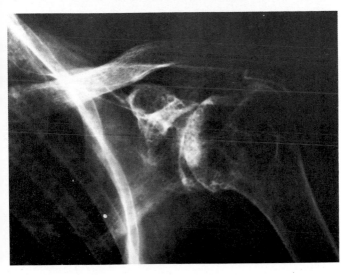

Fig. 2.43 X-rays demonstrate destruction of the head of the humerus and subluxation of the joint; movement is restricted and the patient is unable to lift his arm to comb his hair.

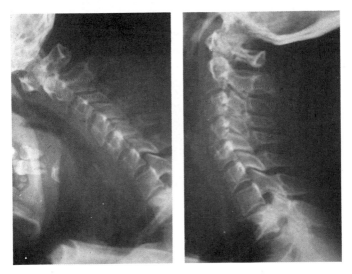

Fig. 2.44 Atlanto-axial RA may lead to subluxation of the atlas, best seen by comparing flexed and extended neck X-rays. If the odontoid peg is difficult to visualise, the slip may be apparent by a change in the relative positions of the two upper spinous processes. Such patients must be treated with great care during intubation for surgery and may need to wear a collar. Surgical fusion may be required to prevent cord compression.

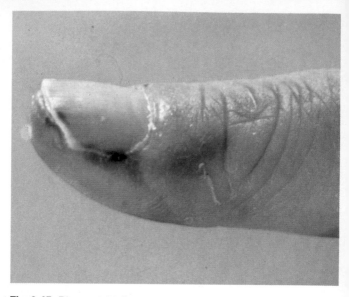

Fig. 2.45 Rheumatoid disease may produce a vasculitis. This type with periungual infarctions is generally mild and may be associated with the use of steroids.

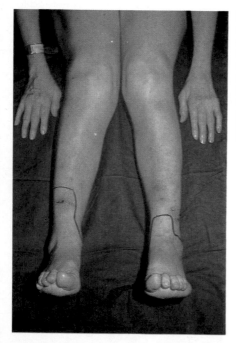

Fig. 2.46 More severe vasculitis of the skin produces painful ulcers and may accompany either a mononeuritis multiplex or a distal neuropathy: this patient has extensive numbness of the lower legs.

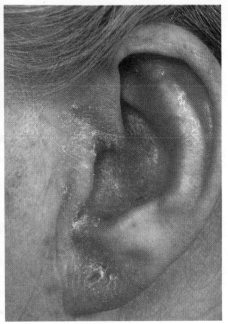

Fig. 2.47 Gold therapy may induce prolonged remission in individual patients although its long-term benefit is difficult to demonstrate in RA as a whole. Its use is limited by side-effects; proteinuria, bone marrow suppression and skin rashes. Routine checks are mandatory. This patient developed a widespread eczematous rash and subsequently flared on stopping the treatment. Rarely, life-threatening exfoliative dermatitis develops, but mild rashes may be managed with a dose reduction.

Patient's Name. J.A. Smith
Number... 235624
Date of Birth. 11/8/50

Gold Treatment Record Card

Date	Injection dose	Total dose	Skin	Urine	Blood	Comments
1/2/82	5mg	5mg	✓	✓	✓	
8/2/82	50mg	55mg	✓	✓	✓	CONTINUE 50mg WEEKLY
15/2/82	50mg	105mg	✓	✓	✓	
22/2/82	50mg	155mg	✓	✓	✓	
1/3/82	50mg	205mg	✓	✓	✓	
8/3/82	50mg	255mg	✓	✓	✓	
15/3/82	50mg	305mg	✓	✓	✓	
22/3/82	50mg	355mg	RASH			STOP GOLD TREATMENT

Fig. 2.48 Regular checks for side effects on long-term therapy are best ensured by the provision of a gold treatment card or other aides memoires. Patients on cytotoxic therapy should be carefully monitored and those on hydroxychloroquine require regular ophthalmological tests.

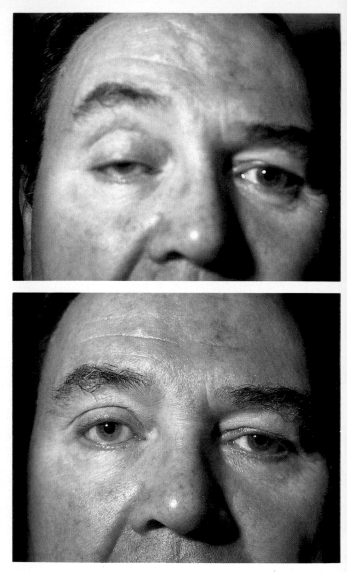

Fig. 2.49 D-Penicillamine produces certain specific side effects. The commonest is an unpleasant taste in the mouth or loss of taste. This is usually transient but may cause discontinuation. Although rare, other side effects with gold or D-Penicillamine do arise – careful follow-up and a high index of suspicion are essential. This patient developed myasthenia gravis on D-Penicillamine: ptosis before (top) and after (bottom) edrophonium. The patient's eye returned to normal, but his arthritis flared after stopping the drug.

41

In addition to the features illustrated previously (nodules, vasculitis and neuropathy) and the more general indicators of systemic disease such as fatigue, malaise and anaemia, rheumatoid disease may affect the eye (episcleritis and occasionally scleromalacia perforans) or the lung (pleural effusions, intrapulmonary nodules or occasionally basal fibrosis). Generalised lymphadenopathy is occasionally seen – the histological changes are non-specific.

Sjögrens syndrome is quite commonly associated with RA and may be very distressing. It is characterised by a dry mouth due to reduced salivary secretions, and dry, gritty eyes (keratoconjunctivitis sicca) caused by reduced tear production. Artificial tears and measures to increase salivation are of some value.

Felty's syndrome with splenomegaly, neutropenia and often leg ulceration is occasionally seen in long-standing RA and is difficult to manage. The neutropenia is multifactorial: hypersplenism, specific antineutrophil antibodies and/or bone marrow precursor suppression may be found

The kidneys are almost never affected by the rheumatoid process, being more commonly damaged by drugs (analgesics, gold or D-penicillamine). Rarely, amyloidosis may lead to proteinuria.

Despite the lack of satisfactory drugs, rheumatoid arthritis is a disease which rarely kills the patient, although side effects from drugs may occasionally be fatal. Thus, in general, it is a disease with which both the patient and the doctor have to come to terms. Properly managed, with attention to regular monitoring and to the wider problems and needs of the patient, he or she should be able to remain an active and productive member of society. Many demonstrate remarkable forbearance and good humour despite their disabilities and fortunately only a small proportion advance progressively towards serious disability.

Pain in the neck, shoulders and arms

The diagnosis of pain in the upper limb is confusing because of the tendency for pain to radiate distally. Careful history-taking and examination are essential if the pattern of pain, exacerbating and alleviating movements, associated neurological symptoms, and signs of a generalised disease are to be elicited.

Radiological changes of cervical spondylosis are common with increasing age but their detection does not explain pain in the neck, arm or shoulder unless there is additional clinical evidence relating it to cervical disease. The neck may be stiff or may show restriction of certain movements and pain may be felt at the extremes of movement. Nerve root irritation due to a disc protrusion or to osteophytic encroachment on the root canal may either produce deep, boring, proximal pain or distal lancinating pain radiating to the lower arm. The latter is frequently associated with paraesthesia and there may be localised neurological signs.

The shoulder has the most comprehensive range of movement of any joint in the body. This is achieved by a complicated musculo-tendinous mechanism which both effects movements and stabilises the joint. Integrity of this mechanism is essential for proper function of the joint; the bony structures themselves providing minimal stability. Pain originating in the shoulder is rarely felt proximal to the shoulder strap line, although if severe there may be secondary painful spasms in the trapezius muscle. Severe shoulder pain may occasionally radiate as far as the wrist. A careful history of the site and nature of reported pain, and examination of the range of movements and any associated pain are often sufficient to localise the lesion. Pain in the shoulder may originate from the neck, from the apex of the lung, from the thoracic outlet, from myocardial disease or from pleural or peritoneal disease affecting the diaphragm. Bilateral shoulder pain usually with severe morning stiffness may be the presenting feature of polymyalgia rheumatica.

The commonest cause of elbow pain is epicondylitis: tennis, or occasionally golfer's, elbow. The joint may be involved in a polyarthritis, particularly rheumatoid arthritis, or may be the site of infective arthritis. Pain in the hand may originate from a proximal lesion or may be due to local factors such as arthritis, tenosynovitis or local nerve entrapment.

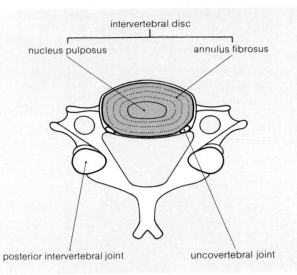

Fig. 3.1 The intervertebral disc comprises an outer fibro-elastic mesh of fibres (the annulus fibrosus) enclosing the gel of the nucleus pulposus. This combination enables the disc to act as a shock absorber and to permit the distortion which facilitates spinal movements.

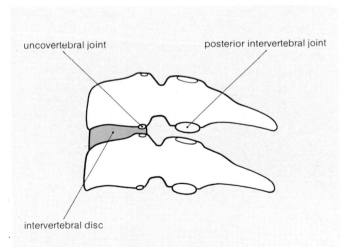

Fig. 3.2 The cervical spine is the most freely mobile part of the vertebral column. In the adult two pairs of synovial joints between adjacent cervical vertebrae allow gliding movements to occur. The top two cervical vertebrae are modified and permit rotation of the head.

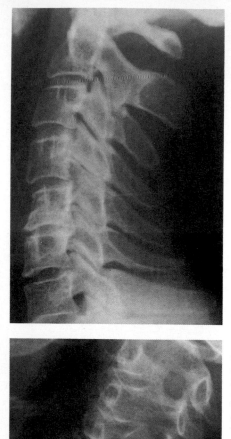

Fig. 3.3 As the disc ages, its water content decreases, the annulus loses its elasticity and the disc becomes less efficient. Disc degeneration is seen on X-rays as a reduction of intervertebral distance and occurs most commonly, as here, in the lower cervical spine (C5-6). This is frequently asymptomatic.

Fig. 3.4 Disc degeneration leads to stressing of the zygapophyseal and intervertebral joints which undergo degenerative changes with bone sclerosis and osteophyte formation. Osteophyte encroachment on the root canal which can be visualised on oblique X-rays (here C6-7), may lead to nerve root symptoms and signs.

Root	Level	Reduced Reflex	Reduced Power
C5	C4-5	Biceps	Shoulder
C6	C5-6	Biceps Brachio-radialis	Biceps Wrist extensors
C7	C6-7	Triceps	Triceps
C8	C7-T1	Triceps	Intrinsics of hand

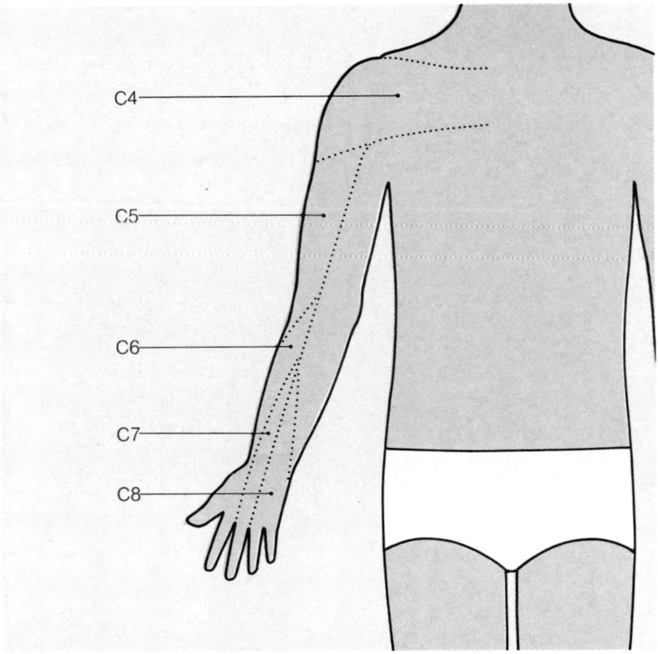

Fig. 3.5 Nerve root irritation, either by an acute disc prolapse or due to spondylosis, may produce these specific symptoms and signs (top). The distribution of paraesthesia and lancinating pain may also localise the lesion (bottom) but the more constant deep pain is less specific.

46

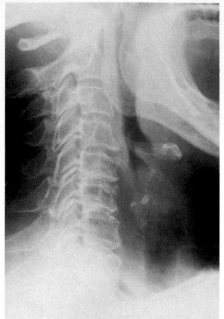

Fig. 3.6 More advanced spondylosis, as illustrated, may produce stiffness but little pain. In general, pain due to cervical spondylosis requires analgesia, local warmth and other measures to reduce muscle spasm. A soft collar may help in the acute phase. Physiotherapy plays an important part in alleviating pain and in giving preventative advice and exercises.

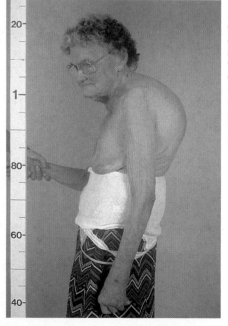

Fig. 3.7 Similar pain is often associated with the development of a dorsal kyphosis, as in this elderly lady with senile osteoporosis. In such cases, postural correction is not possible. Local physiotherapy may produce temporary comfort and relief.

47

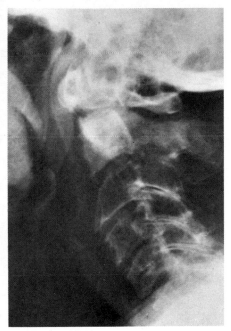

Fig. 3.8 Neck pain is a feature of rheumatoid arthritis (see Fig. 2.44). A central cervical disc prolapse or a secondary deposit in a cervical vertebra may also produce cord compression requiring urgent neurosurgical referral. Here, a patient with cervical spondylosis also has Paget's disease of C2 with typical trabeculae and bone enlargement.

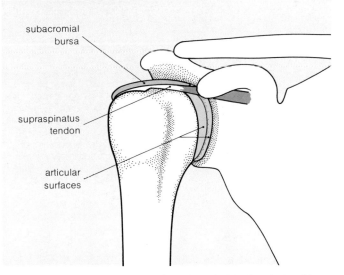

subacromial bursa

supraspinatus tendon

articular surfaces

Fig. 3.9 The complex structure of the shoulder ideally suits its wide range of movements. There are three main synovial joints and in addition the subacromial structures act as a joint, as does the scapula, rotating on the chest wall.

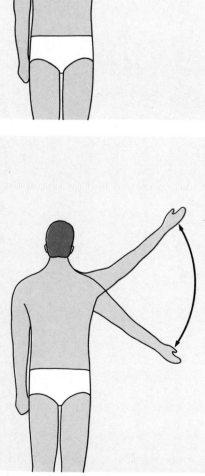
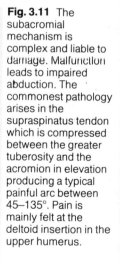

Fig. 3.10 The acromioclavicular joint produces pain which is typically felt over the top of the shoulder and is exacerbated by extreme elevation or adduction in internal rotation (reaching behind the back). If local anaesthetic injection into the joint reduces pain, it is of diagnostic value.

Fig. 3.11 The subacromial mechanism is complex and liable to damage. Malfunction leads to impaired abduction. The commonest pathology arises in the supraspinatus tendon which is compressed between the greater tuberosity and the acromion in elevation producing a typical painful arc between 45–135°. Pain is mainly felt at the deltoid insertion in the upper humerus.

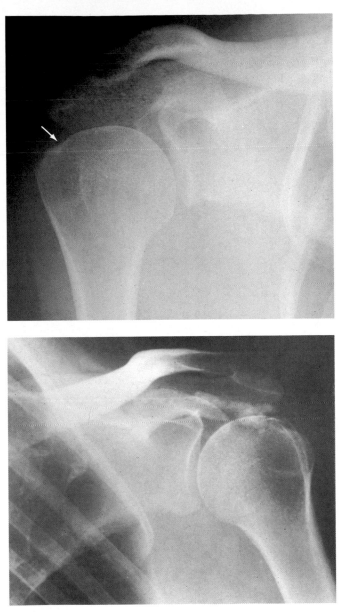

Fig. 3.12 Localised calcification in the supraspinatus tendon probably reflects an old lesion (top), but more severe pain and restriction of movement may be associated with an acute deposition of crystals in the region of the subacromial bursa (bottom). An injection with local anaesthetic and a corticosteroid is indicated.

50

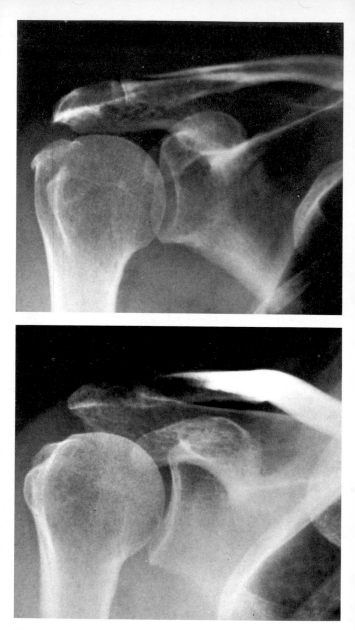

Fig. 3.13 With severe prolonged tendon inflammation, degenerative cystic sclerosis and osteophytes may develop (top). Severe reduction of movement develops and secondary muscle atrophy is common. The lower X-ray is normal.

51

<u>Adhesive capsulitis</u> (frozen shoulder) is a syndrome seen in the 40–60 year old and is typified by spontaneous gradual onset of pain and stiffness in one shoulder. At first the pain is particularly troublesome at night, but over a few weeks gradually subsides. The stiffness continues to increase for several months, however, until all movements are grossly reduced, before abating spontaneously about 12–18 months after onset. Investigations are all normal although arthrography reveals constriction of the joint capsule and a reduced joint volume. The aetiology is unknown. Once the pain has subsided, recovery of movement is probably best accelerated by manipulation under anaesthetic followed by intensive physiotherapy. By such means the course may be reduced from 18 months to 18 weeks.

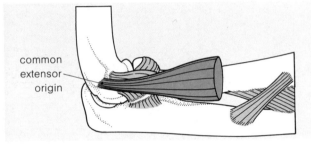

Fig. 3.14 Tennis elbow is a common cause of pain at the elbow and in the upper forearm, arising from the common origin of the wrist extensors at the lateral epicondyle. Pain is exacerbated by carrying a bag and other powerful contractions of the wrist extensors and there is marked tenderness localised at the lateral epicondyle. Treatment is rest and injection of a corticosteroid and local anaesthetic into the most tender area. This may initially exacerbate the pain.

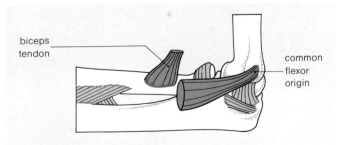

Fig. 3.15 Golfer's elbow is a similar and less common lesion affecting the common flexor origin at the medial epicondyle. Treatment is as for tennis elbow but care should be taken because of the proximity of the ulnar nerve to the medial epicondyle.

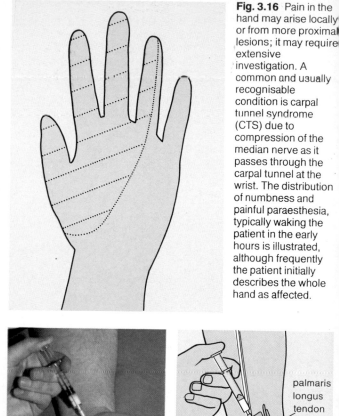

Fig. 3.16 Pain in the hand may arise locally or from more proximal lesions; it may require extensive investigation. A common and usually recognisable condition is carpal tunnel syndrome (CTS) due to compression of the median nerve as it passes through the carpal tunnel at the wrist. The distribution of numbness and painful paraesthesia, typically waking the patient in the early hours is illustrated, although frequently the patient initially describes the whole hand as affected.

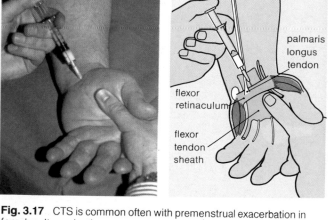

palmaris longus tendon

flexor retinaculum

flexor tendon sheath

Fig. 3.17 CTS is common often with premenstrual exacerbation in females. It may be the presentation of polyarthritis (early RA) or rarely myxoedema, or may follow a fracture of the wrist. Occasionally nerve conduction studies may be necessary to establish the diagnosis. Classical cases can be treated by locally injected corticosteroid – *local anaesthetic should only be used on the skin. Technique:* The needle is introduced at 45° at the distal wrist crease to the radial side of palmaris longus tendon or, in its absence, between flexor carpi radialis and flexor digitorum sublimis. Rarely, surgical release is necessary.

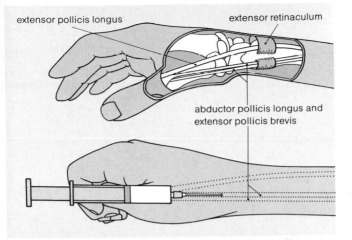

Fig. 3.18 De Quervain's tenosynovitis (affecting the sheath of abductor pollicis longus and extensor pollicis brevis) produces pain and tenderness over the radial styloid which is exacerbated by forced flexion of the thumb into the palm. Treatment is by local injection of local anaesthetic and corticosteroid into the inflamed tendon sheath using the technique illustrated.

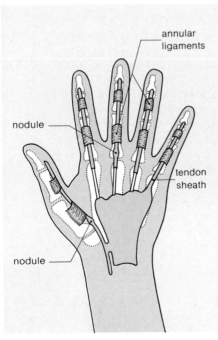

Fig. 3.19 Nodular swelling of the flexor tendons of the fingers and thumbs may occur alone or as part of RA. Initially asymptomatic, they may lead to 'triggering' of the finger involved; the patient often awakens with the digit flexed and has to force it to extend. This may become painful or occasionally impossible. Local injection of local anaesthetic and corticosteroid into the sheath is usually very effective – rarely surgery is indicated.

Pain in the lower back and legs

Most people experience low back pain at some time during their lives, but the majority of these episodes are mild and self-limited. Not all patients present to their doctor, but those who do contribute significantly to the total number of days lost from work due to sickness. Although such transient episodes are difficult to diagnose precisely, substantial efforts are now being put into research to define the lesions and to assess their prevention. Many painful complaints of the spinal column and its complex ligments and musculature are almost certainly traumatic in origin and caused by excessive stressing. The spine is a remarkable structure combining weight-bearing functions with flexibility – however, the end result is ideal for neither. Mechanical stresses in the lumbar spine are increased greatly under the loading caused by forward flexion and more so by lifting in the flexed position. Twisting movements under such loading exert considerable torque on the shock-absorbing intervertebral discs and stress the facet joints and ligaments. Ill-advised lifting, poor posture and general lack of muscle tone all contribute to the morbidity of mechanical problems of the spine and are potentially preventable.

Fortunately most of the self-limited episodes resolve rapidly with simple measures such as analgesia and rest. The largest case load presenting to GPs occurs in the sixth and seventh decades and although most patients do not require extensive investigation, such features as persistent or recurrent pain, especially when unrelieved by resting in bed, associated neurological symptoms or signs, or evidence of systemic disease suggest more sinister pathology and indicate that more thorough investigation may be warranted. It is hoped that this section will provide an insight into the diagnosis and management of these important conditions.

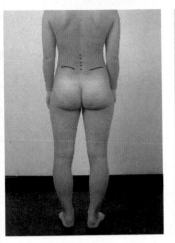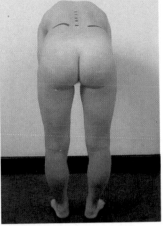

Fig. 4.1 A clear history and thorough examination are essential in all but the most trivial cases of back pain. Particular attention should be paid to trauma, a past history of similar events or a relevant family history. The patient is best examined fully undressed, observation being made of general posture, any asymmetry or pelvic obliquity and scoliosis. Observed from behind the patient is asked to flex forwards as far as possible and return to upright – such movements may exacerbate pain, the site of which should be noted together with any change in a scoliosis and the degree of limitation of flexion. Extension, lateral flexion and rotation should be observed and restriction and pain noted.

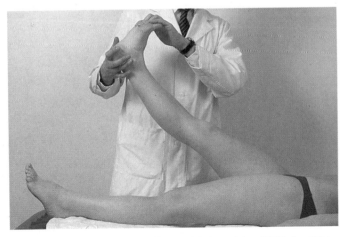

Fig. 4.2 With the patient supine the straight leg raising (SLR) should be measured – if limited and associated with pain radiating down the leg, nerve root compression is suggested. The distribution of sensory loss is recorded, muscle power tested and the reflexes examined. The peripheral pulses should be palpated.

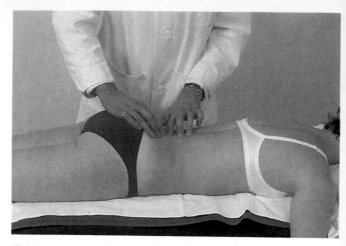

Fig. 4.3 With the patient prone, localised tenderness can be mapped out; this may respond to locally injected corticosteroids and local anaesthetic. Peri-anal (saddle) sensory loss may occur in lesions affecting the cauda equina which in addition to causing back pain are often complicated by urinary retention and bilateral neurological signs in the legs. In such cases urgent neurosurgical referral is indicated. All patients with low back pain should have a rectal and pelvic examination.

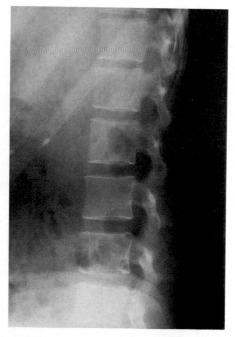

Fig. 4.4 Low back pain may produce postural changes as in this case with extreme loss of lumbar lordosis. No other radiological abnormality was found and the patient did well with general physiotherapeutic measures and postural advice. Sagging posture and increased lordosis may produce low back pain.

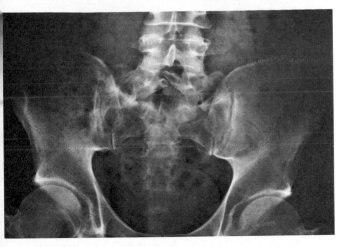

Fig. 4.5 The finding of occult spina bifida is common during X-ray examination of patients for other reasons; its role in the aetiology of low back pain is uncertain although there is some indication that it is associated with an increased incidence of mechanical back problems. It may help the patient to understand why they should be getting pain but care must be taken not to alarm them or induce anxiety. Physiotherapy may be helpful.

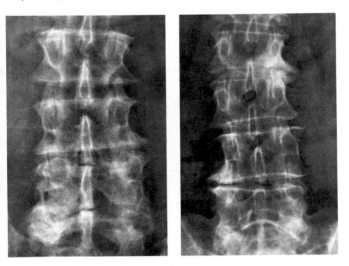

Fig. 4.6 Lumbar spondylosis is common with increasing age and is often asymptomatic as here (left), found during a skeletal survey done for other reasons. The radiologically less severely affected patient on the right had suffered from intermittent low back pain for years and eventually resorted to a corset with some benefit (after other measures had failed). Typical beak-like osteophytes are seen (compare Fig. 4.24).

Disc	Nerve Root	Reduced Reflex	Reduced Power	Pain/Paraesthesia
L3-4	L4	Knee	Knee extension (quadriceps)	Anterolateral thigh and medial calf
L4-5	L5	None	Dorsiflexion of great toe	Lateral calf
L5-S1	S1	Ankle	Plantar flexion (gastrocnemius)	Lateral foot and back of calf

Fig. 4.7 Sciatic pain due to lumbar disc prolapse is usually acute in onset and often follows injury whilst twisting, bending and lifting. The patient may be immobilised by pain in the spine and radiating down one leg. Unilateral paraesthesia are highly suggestive of root compression in such situations. The SLR will be grossly limited and leg pain exacerbated by dorsiflexion of the foot at the extreme of SLR, (sciatic stretch test). Careful examination of neurological signs may locate the lesion.

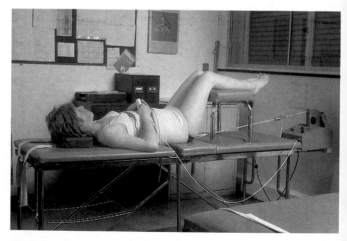

Fig. 4.8 Treatment of an acute disc prolapse is initially bed rest and analgesia followed by physiotherapy when the acute pain has settled. Lumbar traction may help, mainly by relaxing muscular spasm. With persistent pain in-patient care is indicated; complete bed rest at home is often very difficult in practice.

59

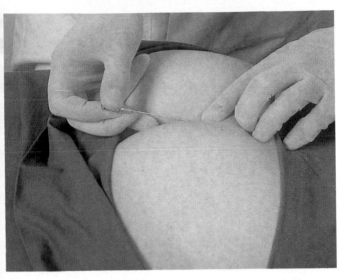

Fig. 4.9 The role of epidural injections of long-acting anaesthetic agents with or without corticosteroids is controversial in acute disc prolapse, although some patients do experience rapid pain relief which may enable them to avoid time off work. The epidural can usually be satisfactorily carried out by a sacral approach (as illustrated) except in patients with high lesions, when a lumbar approach is best. The technique requires practice.

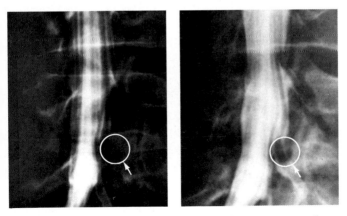

Fig. 4.10 In persistent cases who do not respond to more conservative measures, or when neurological signs are gross, a surgical opinion should be sought and radiculography performed. Although a safe procedure, this is generally not performed unless surgery is being actively considered. In this patient there was occlusion of the left L5 root sheath (left) which was completely free in a follow up study for recurrent pain (right).

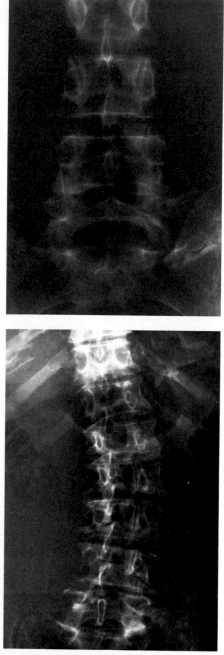

Fig. 4.11 The previous patient was found to have hemisacralisation of his fifth lumbar vertebra which increases the stresses at L4-5 and is associated with an increased incidence of disc prolapse at this level. Laminectomy itself may produce mild back pain post-operatively and the patient should be warned of this before surgery is undertaken.

Fig. 4.12 Nerve root compression in older patients may be due to root canal stenosis associated with spondylosis and the formation of osteophytes at the posterolateral vertebral margin and on the facet joints. This patient with a scoliosis showed this picture with acute pain precipitated by an L4-5 disc prolapse; she responded well to canal decompression. Occasionally a picture of root pain brought on by exercise occurs: root claudication.

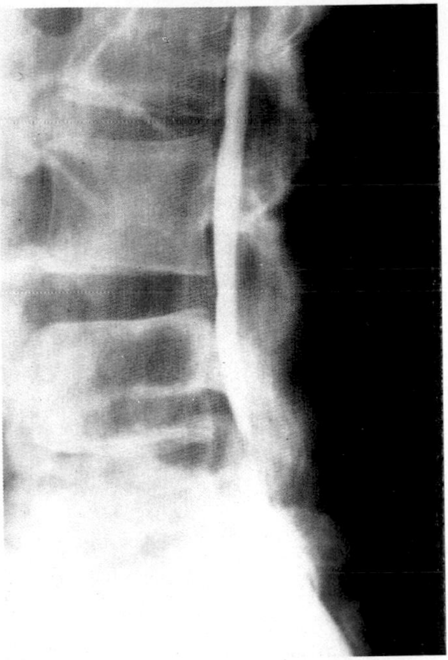

Fig. 4.13 Some patients have congenitally narrowed spinal canals demonstrated here by myelography. Such patients are at greater risk of neurological damage due to posterior osteophyte formation or acute central disc prolapse (here L4-5). They may also develop bilateral symptoms of cauda equina claudication. Leg pulses are usually normal. Surgical decompression is indicated.

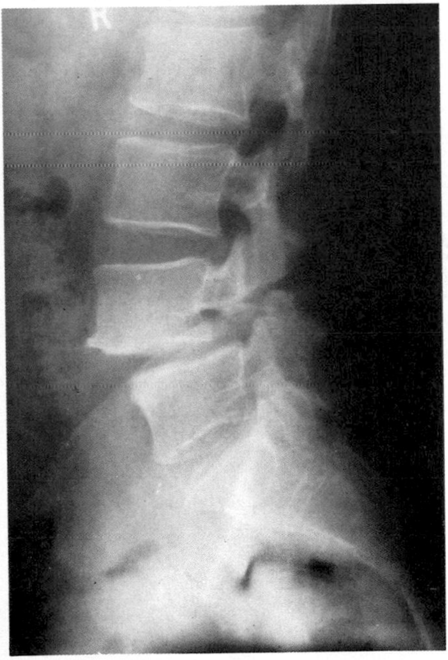

Fig. 4.14 A spondylolisthesis may exacerbate canal narrowing but is frequently asymptomatic. The degree of slip is assessed according to the percentage of the vertebral body exposed. Unstable spondylolistheses may present with severe back and leg symptoms and warrant surgical stabilisation. In the stable case intermittent use of a corset may suffice.

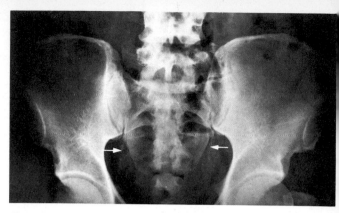

Fig. 4.15 Leg pain due to true claudication of the calf or other muscles quite commonly presents to the rheumatology clinic; in the older patient the foot, popliteal and femoral pulses should be examined and if necessary Doppler flow studies arranged. This 34 year old, poorly controlled diabetic presented with claudication at 50 yards; arterial calcification is apparent in the pelvic vessels.

Patients with generalised osteoarthritis often complain of difficulty in walking which is frequently due to painful hips and unstable knees; occasionally such cases are however due to paraparesis developing in association with cord compression due to cervical spondylosis or cauda equina compression due to lumbar disease. All such patients require a careful neurological examination.

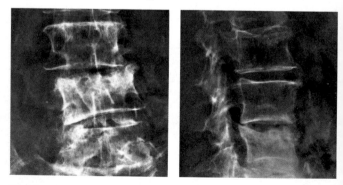

Fig. 4.16 Acute pain in the lumbar or thoracic spine, often after a fall or jarring, is seen in postmenopausal women and occasionally in elderly men due to osteoporotic collapse of a vertebra, as here. The most important differential diagnoses are collapse due to a primary or secondary tumour in the vertebra or associated with an infective lesion. In osteoporotic collapse the vertebral cortices are fractured but intact. Bed rest, analgesia and support in a corset are needed in the acute episode.

63

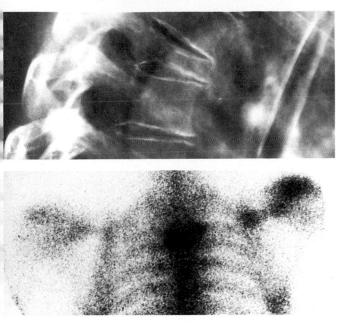

Fig. 4.17 By contrast, in collapse due to myelomatous or secondary deposits there is often loss of definition of part of the cortical margins of the affected vertebra. If the lesion is suspicious, other investigations must be undertaken. In this patient with a past history of mastectomy, a bone scan confirmed further deposits in the right shoulder. The painful vertebral collapse was treated by local radiotherapy.

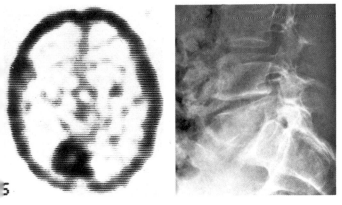

Fig. 4.18 Other investigations may include examination of blood or urine for myeloma protein, bronchoscopy or brain scanning. In this case, the patient presented with pain due to collapse of L5 He was also confused because of the cerebral secondary deposit. Direct biopsy of the fifth lumbar vertebra confirmed the primary as bronchial in origin.

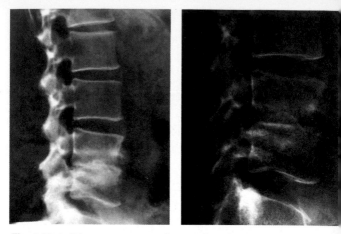

Fig. 4.19 In this case a young male recently arrived from the Indian sub-continent presented with back pain, fever and weight loss. In addition to the clues from his general illness the X-rays show gross loss of the L4-5 disc space together with destruction of the cortical margins of *both* adjacent vertebrae. Biopsy of the lesion under radiological control yielded tubercle bacilli and he was started on therapy for 18 months; in the second X-ray healing has occurred and he was already back at work.

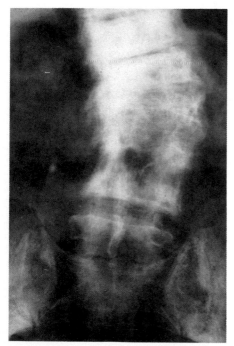

Fig. 4.20 Sclerosis of vertebrae or of the sacral and iliac bones may be found in patients presenting with back pain. In this case there is clear enlargement of the vertebra as well as sclerosis – a diagnostic feature of Paget's disease. Similar lesions were found elsewhere in the skeleton including the femur; they responded well to *intermittent* courses of calcitonin. (Caution – this therapy is expensive and has a high incidence of side effects. It should be used with circumspection and in intermittent courses.)

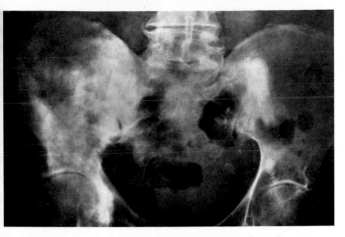

Fig. 4.21 Sclerotic lesions may also occur in metastatic malignancy – most commonly prostatic carcinoma as in this case where the diagnosis was confirmed by a raised acid phosphatase and prostatic biopsy. A bone scan showed widespread deposits. If there is uncertainty diagnostic biopsy of the affected vertebra should be attempted. Pain due to malignancy responds well to local radiotherapy which also reduces the risk of subsequent vertebral collapse.

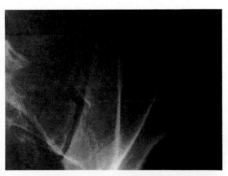

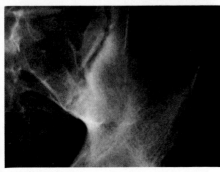

Fig. 4.22 One of the typical features of back pain associated with inflammatory sacro-iliitis is early morning exacerbation associated with severe morning spinal stiffness. This may be seen in patients with ankylosing spondylitis (AS). It is more common in males and usually presents in the twenties or thirties; X-rays may shown no abnormality early on but later the typical changes of sacroiliitis develop with irregularity and patchy sclerosis of the joint margins. Here a coned view of a normal joint (top) is compared with one in AS (bottom). These changes are usually bilateral.

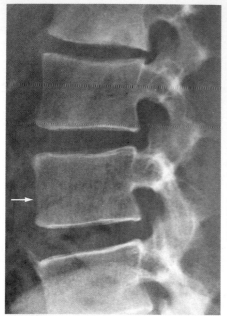

Fig. 4.23 Early vertebral changes in AS include a squaring-off of the anterior vertebral surface, as can be seen in this lumbar vertebra. The intervertebral ligaments involved in the inflammatory process typically heal by ossification, leading to the formation of syndesmophytes which follow the line of the ligaments. Early changes may be localised to the thoracolumbar junction.

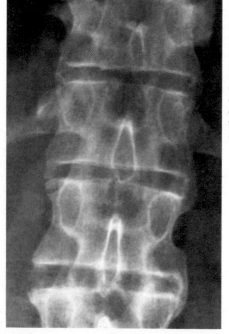

Fig. 4.24 Eventually the disc space becomes bridged by the syndesmophyte; its shape and the preservation of the intervertebral disc distinguish it from a degenerative osteophyte secondary to spondylosis (compare Fig. 4.6).

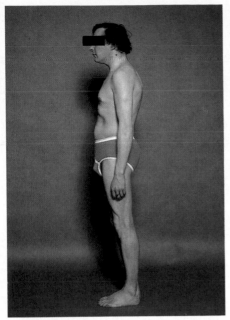

Fig. 4.25 The typical posture of AS develops late in the disease and should be avoidable by analgesia and postural exercises. This young patient is showing early signs with a fixed dorsal kyphosis and bulging abdomen, the latter due to abdominal breathing. Later, hip and knee flexion develop as the kyphosis worsens and the neck becomes hyperextended to facilitate forward vision.

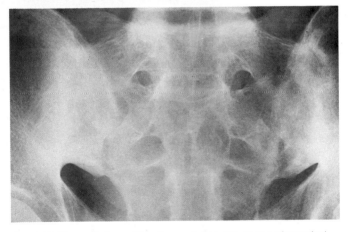

Fig. 4.26 The end stage of the disease is to produce complete spinal fusion (bamboo spine) with ossification of all the ligamentous structures and fusion of the SI joints, as seen here. This is probably prevented by the controlled use of analgesic anti-inflammatory agents during painful flares to allow the patient to exercise vigorously thus maintaining both spinal movement and posture. AS is associated with the genetic histocompatibility marker HLA B27, present in 8% of Caucasian controls, but in 95% of patients with AS. (Tissue typing is not a routine investigation; it is unnecessary in the classical case.)

68

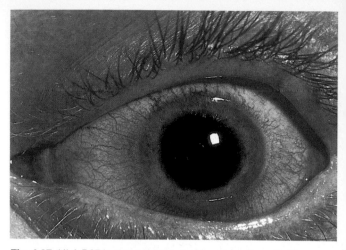

Fig. 4.27 HLA B27 is also associated with certain other arthritic complaints which may be complicated by sacroiliitis – see chapter 6. Such patients may also develop painful acute anterior uveitis with blurring of vision and typical peri-iridial injection associated with distinctive features on slit-lamp examination. Urgent ophthalmological advice is indicated and the response to local steroids and mydriatics is dramatic; relapse is common.

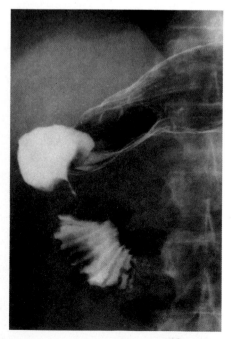

Fig. 4.28 Pain in the lumbar spine and buttocks may be due to disease in the pelvis or in the posterior abdominal wall. The differential diagnosis is wide but includes carcinoma of the pancreas, posterior peptic ulceration, abdominal aneurysm of the aorta and infiltrating pelvic tumours. In such cases computerised axial tomography is often the most rapid diagnostic procedure. Here, a carcinoma of the pancreas is producing concentric narrowing of the duodenum.

In the space available a complete analysis of the management of low back pain is not possible. Physical measures remain the key to the management of many of the mechanical problems, combined with attention to prevention by advice on posture, work and cybernetic design. An attempt has been made to indicate when a surgical referral is necessary and also to demonstrate the importance of a full history and careful examination in deciding how extensively the patient should be investigated. As a general rule, in the younger patient with mechanical low back pain, X-rays are unlikely to be helpful.

The role of the patient's emotional state and of stress in the aetiology of low back pain is controversial and in general it is best to assume that there is always an underlying physical lesion although this is often mild. Depression, anxiety and stress may well modify the patient's ability to cope with pain and, by inducing muscle tension, may compound the problem. Such matters must be discussed with the patient with great care and tact if the physician is to maintain his rapport. Alienation from traditional medicine is the commonest cause of patients turning in desperation to various types of fringe medicine which vary from helpful to positively dangerous.

Acute monoarthritis

The sudden onset of inflammation in one joint is typical of several different types of arthritis. The most striking cases are usually those of crystal synovitis caused by either uric acid crystals (gout) or calcium pyrophosphate (pseudogout). In such cases the cardinal signs of inflammation are all present; redness, swelling, heat, pain and loss of function. Gout of the great toe MTP joint (podalgia) is often so painful that even the weight of a bed sheet is unbearable. Similarly, florid signs are also seen with an acute haemarthrosis which may occur in patients with a bleeding diathesis or occasionally in a joint with pre-existing OA. A more common cause of sudden swelling and increase of pain in an osteoarthritic joint is so-called traumatic synovitis; this may be associated with inflammation due to crystals of calcium hydroxyapatite. Mention has already been made of infective arthritis as the cause of an acute monoarticular flare in a patient with RA (page 31). Infection may also affect previously normal joints producing an acute arthritis in most cases, and with an associated fever and leukocytosis. The latter features may be seen in more acute cases of gout and pseudogout, however, and are thus not diagnostic.

The essential diagnostic procedure in all cases is to attempt to aspirate the joint and then to *immediately* examine the fluid both macro- and microscopically: treatment should be delayed until this has been done in all but exceptional cases. The sample should be cultured routinely and when indicated also for gonococci and/or *Mycobacterium tuberculosis*. A full physical examination is essential and blood tests, X-rays and culture of samples from other sites may also be necessary.

When there is a clear history of a twisting injury and/or locking (inability to fully extend or flex the joint), cartilage damage, loose bodies or fracture must also enter the differential diagnosis. Most forms of polyarthritis present occasionally in one joint and may also need to be excluded.

With careful diagnosis and correct treatment in acute crystal synovitis and in other causes of acute monoarthritis, rapid symptomatic improvement is usual and a complete cure is often achieved.

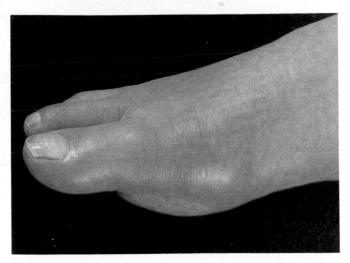

Fig. 5.1 Acute podalgia caused by urate synovitis is so painful and the clinical appearances are so typical that diagnosis is rarely a problem, although an infected bunion may occasionally have a similar appearance. Joint aspiration may be difficult from small joints and treatment can be started with non-steroidal anti-inflammatory drugs whilst the result of a confirmatory serum urate level is awaited.

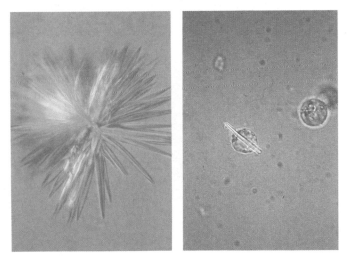

Fig. 5.2 The typical needle-shaped urate crystals can be identified under polarising light when they show strongly negative birefringence. Polymorphs containing the crystals are often seen; it is failure to digest the crystals which leads to the release of pro-inflammatory substances. Colchicine is now less commonly used in acute gout, but it is cheap; it acts by preventing polymorphs from ingesting the crystals.

Causes of hyperuricaemia and gout

Primary

Genetic factors, race etc.

Secondary

Starvation eg. postoperative

Obesity

High alcohol intake

Thiazide diuretic therapy

Changes in renal function

Increase in nucleoprotein turnover —psoriasis
—leukaemias
—cytotoxic therapy

Lead poisoning (saturnine gout)

Fig. 5.3 Gout may affect any joint and may also present as a polyarticular onset with fever and a leukocytosis. This is more common now that thiazide diuretics are so widely used; these impair renal handling of urate. Premenopausal women rarely suffer gout but thiazides seem to be leading to an increased incidence in elderly women. Other factors predisposing to hyperuricaemia and thus to acute gout are listed above.

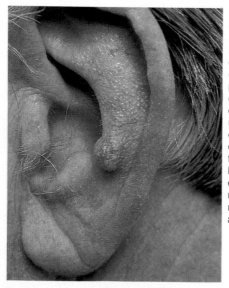

Fig. 5.4 Although the detection of uric acid crystals or of a raised serum urate is diagnostic, certain clinical features may point to the diagnosis of gout; tophaceous deposits of crystalline uric acid may be found commonly in the pinna of the ear or on the fingers. A family history of gout may be elicited especially in male patients or they may describe typical attacks in the past.

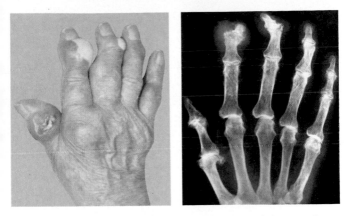

Fig. 5.5 Hyperuricaemia may lead to a different type of picture such as in this elderly lady who has visible tophi on her fingers associated with cystic changes in adjacent joints. The tophaceous deposits show up as a typical 'halo' on the X-ray; they can thus be distinguished from the more radio-dense deposits of calcinosis such as are seen in scleroderma.

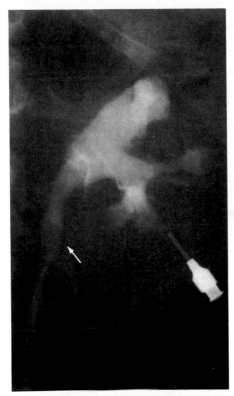

Fig. 5.6 Renal damage may be found in patients presenting with gout or with tophi. It may be the cause of the hyperuricaemia as, for example, in the type of gout associated with chronic lead poisoning (saturnine gout), or may be a result of it. Some patients present with renal colic due to radiolucent uric acid stones.

Acute gout should be treated with non-steroidal-anti-inflammatory drugs (NSAIDs) such as indomethacin: 100mg, is given immediately, then 50mg three times daily for a few days with the dose tailing off over several weeks. Colchicine is given in a dose of 1mg, then $500\mu g$ three hourly for nine hours and finally $500\mu g$ three times a day. Diarrhoea is an unpleasant side-effect. Recurrent gout, tophaceous gout or occasionally severe asymptomatic hyperuricaemia all need treatment with the xanthine oxidase inhibitor, allopurinol, which blocks uric acid production. The usual dose is 100 - 400mg daily. Uricosuric agents are useful in tophaceous gout usually as an adjunct to allopurinol, but should not be used in the presence of renal damage or in patients with urate renal stones. Allopurinol or uricosuric treatment should always be started under a cover of an NSAID for the first eight weeks as they may precipitate acute gouty attacks.

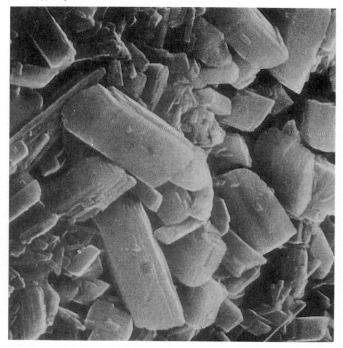

Fig. 5.7 Pseudogout most commonly affects the knees and presents as acute pain and swelling; the diagnosis is confirmed by the finding of triclinic crystals of calcium pyrophosphate in the aspirate, seen here under the electron microscope. They are weakly positively birefringent under polarising light. Treatment is with NSAIDs.

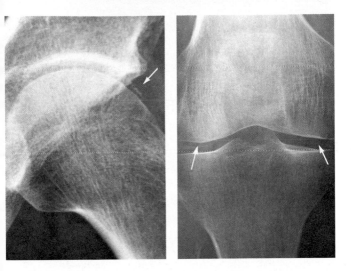

Fig. 5.8 Pseudogout is commonly seen in joints which show the radiological changes of chondrocalcinosis. This patient presented with pseudogout and showed chrondrocalcinosis on his hip and knee X-rays. Such findings should suggest a predisposing disease such as haemochromatosis or hypothyroidism or, as in this case, hyperparathyroidism. The chondrocalcinosis will usually resolve with treatment of the underlying disease. Widespread chondrocalcinosis is also associated with a more chronic and destructive arthritis which resembles OA but in which there is often a prominent inflammatory component.

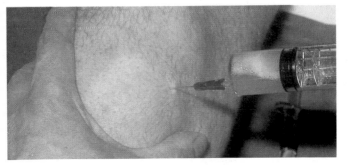

Fig. 5.9 An acutely infected joint is usually associated with systemic malaise, fever and a leukocytosis, although this is also seen in acute gout and pseudogout. The management of a suspected infected joint is to aspirate fluid and send it immediately for staining and culture (see also page 31). A stained film will usually suggest the best antibiotic therapy until sensitivities are available. Rarely antibiotic therapy may need to be started without such findings and in such cases bacterilogical advice should be sought. *Antibiotic therapy should always be delayed until blood and other cultures have been obtained.*

76

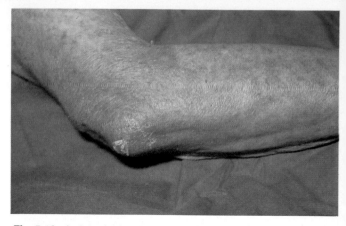

Fig. 5.10 An infective bursitis, here of the olecranon bursa and leading to septicaemia, may at first glance mimic the appearances of an infective arthritis, although it is unusual for such severe limitation of passive joint movement to be produced. The bursa should be aspirated and the fluid examined immediately. A much shorter course of antibiotics is needed in such cases rather than the two to three months usually recommended for infective arthritis.

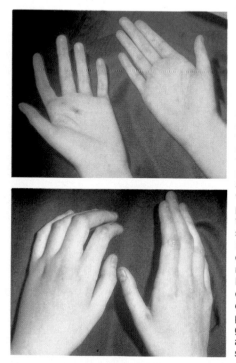

Fig. 5.11
Gonococcal arthritis is now relatively common and may present in symptomatic or asymptomatic patients (female or male). The appearance may be an acute monoarthritis, in which case organisms are often obtained from the aspirate, or more commonly an arthritis of the ankle or wrist associated with a pustular rash and tenosynovitis, as is seen in this patient. In such cases, organisms are usually not found in the joint. Expert advice and contact tracing are essential for all patients with gonorrhoea. They may also have NSU or syphilis.

Synovial fluid examination

Appearance		
	Clear	OA Sero-negative arthritis
	Cloudy	RA Crystal synovitis
	Purulent	Infection

Cell count (using EDTA)	High cell count (>50,000) Predominance of polymorphs	Crystal synovitis Infection

Gram stain and culture	Identification of infective organism Choice of antibiotic

Microscopy under polarised light	Identification of crystals

Fig. 5.12 The key to the diagnosis of an acute monoarthritis in particular is to obtain a sample of synovial fluid and to ensure that if possible it is examined immediately for both organisms and crystals. Joint aspiration is not difficult but requires some practice (see Fig. 2.30). Most rheumatologists will see such cases urgently.

Arthritis affecting a few joints (asymmetrical, pauciarticular arthritis)

Just as certain types of arthritis typically present as either an acute peripheral symmetrical polyarthritis or as an acute monoarthritis, so there is a further group which presents with a picture of asymmetrical joint involvement usually limited to a few joints (pauciarticular arthritis). This group includes the so-called sero-negative arthritides (that is, negative for IgM rheumatoid factor) in which important diagnostic clues can often be obtained from a careful clinical history and examination; most of these cases are associated with other diseases such as psoriasis, non-specific urethritis or certain types of dysentery, chronic inflammatory bowel disease or the typical back pain and stiffness of ankylosing spondylitis (AS). There may be a past history of acute anterior uveitis or a family history of similar arthritis or of one of the associated diseases. Although the inheritance is not clear, there is a wide overlap of the various conditions both clinically and in blood relatives. Thus nail dystrophy is seen in Reiter's syndrome and psoriasis, and the histology of keratoderma blennorrhagica is identical to that of pustular psoriasis. A patient with psoriatic arthritis may also develop Crohn's disease or ulcerative colitis, or may have relatives with one of these conditions.

Over 95% of AS patients carry the genetic histocompatibility antigen HLA B27 which is present in only 8% of a normal Caucasian population. Its incidence is also raised in patients with psoriasis and Reiter's disease, especially those with associated sacroiliitis. Although the significance of this finding is not clear it seems that Reiter's disease and AS may be reactive arthritides to *Chlamydia trachomatis* and *Klebsiella* spp. respectively, in the same way that rheumatic fever is to Lancefield group A β-haemolytic streptococci. The mechanism underlying the disease manifestations may thus be one of cross-reactivity between antibodies directed against the infective organism and host cell surface antigens.

This complicated group of arthritic conditions cannot be completely dealt with in the space available, but it is hoped that this may help the non-specialist practitioner to make the appropriate diagnosis. Most of these types of arthritis carry a relatively better prognosis than that of rheumatoid arthritis although most follow a chronic, relapsing and remitting course.

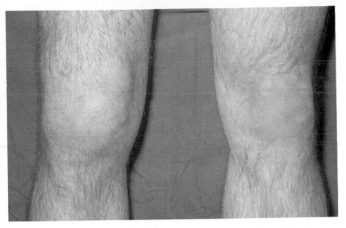

Fig. 6.1 Sexually acquired reactive arthritis presents typically in the young male as an acute arthritis affecting knees, ankles and feet. There is often florid synovial thickening and an effusion. Occasionally an acute monoarticular onset may mimic gout. In the male, urethritis is usually symptomatic with a slight to moderate, clear or purulent discharge. In women, non-specific urethritis, vaginitis and cervicitis associated with arthritis are less common but increasingly recognised. A similar arthritic picture may also follow certain types of dysentery.

Gonorrhoea (see Fig. 5.11) and non-specific urethritis may coexist, the NSU only being diagnosable after the former has been treated with penicillin. Serological tests for syphilis should also be performed. All such cases require the expert advice of a specialist in genito-urinary medicine who will also arrange contact tracing if necessary.

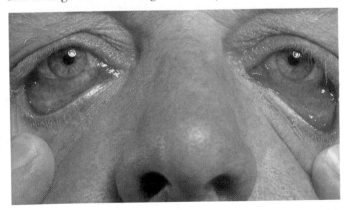

Fig. 6.2 In the classical case, in addition to urethritis and arthritis, a mild conjunctivitis is also present; this triad is called Reiter's disease. A few patients later develop anterior uveitis.

80

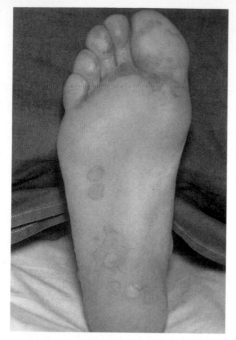

Fig. 6.3 Lesions of the soles and palms also occur. They are initially pustular as shown in this patient but may become confluent and scaly (keratoderma blennorrhagica). These lesions are clinically identical to pustular psoriasis and may be associated with dystrophic nail changes.

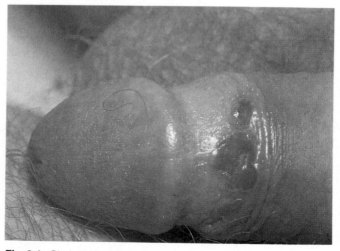

Fig. 6.4 Circinate balanitis is present in many Reiter's cases. In the uncircumcised male it appears as painless moist ulceration of the glans or undersurface of the prepuce and in the circumcised as more scaly lesions. Like the arthritis and keratoderma, balanitis may persist or relapse and remit after the urethritis has been successfully treated with tetracycline.

81

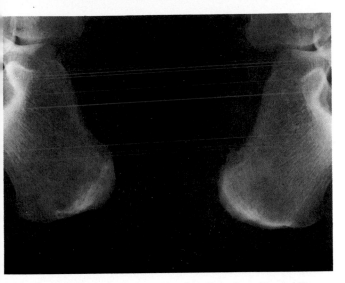

Fig. 6.5 Pain under the heel or at the site of insertion of the Achilles tendon is sufficiently common in reactive arthritis to place this diagnosis top of the differential list in patients with associated arthritis. Radiological changes of 'fluffy' plantar spurs (right) and/or erosions at the insertion of the Achilles tendon into the calcaneum are seen.

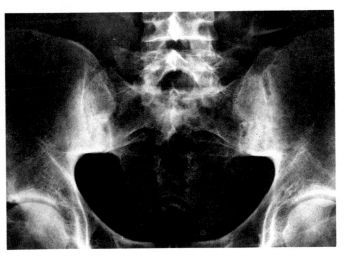

Fig. 6.6 Sacroiliitis may occur in patients with urethritis, or after dysentery. Some of these patients progress to spinal calcification identical to that of ankylosing spondylitis. AS itself (see pages 66–69) may however also present with a peripheral arthritis and may be difficult to distinguish unless a full history is taken and genital examination is carried out.

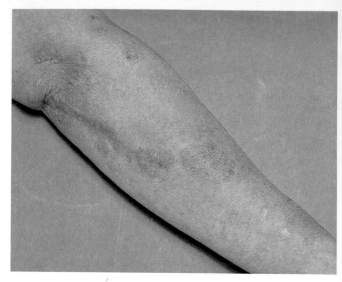

Fig. 6.7 Psoriasis (Ps) typically comprises patchy, red, raised lesions particularly over the elbows and knees. It can be extensive or very localised, for example in the scalp or natal cleft, and may be easily missed. Various patterns of sero-negative arthritis occur in patients with psoriasis; most have a better prognosis than classical RA.

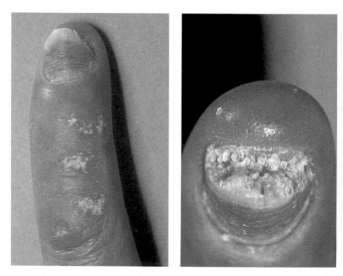

Fig. 6.8 The most benign form of psoriatic arthritis involves the DIP joints. Usually typical changes are present in the adjacent nail; pitting and lifting of the nail from its bed (onycholysis) (left). Occasionally the dystrophy can be more distressing than the arthritis (right).

Arthritis and psoriasis

1. DIP joint involvement* ⎤
                            ⎥ 'Typical'
2. Arthritis mutilans (rare) ⎦

3. Asymmetrical wrists, knees and ankles

4. Rheumatoid-like distribution –
   rheumatoid factor negative

5. Sacroiliitis/ankylosing spondylitis*

6. Coincidental sero-positive RA, or OA

* May coexist with other types

Fig. 6.9 The various types of patterns of psoriatic arthritis are listed above. Both RA and Ps are common and may coexist but there is a rheumatoid-like sero-negative arthritis seen in patients with Ps which does not usually produce severe disability. In most cases NSAIDs control the symptoms during flares but some clinicians advocate the use of gold in progressive cases.

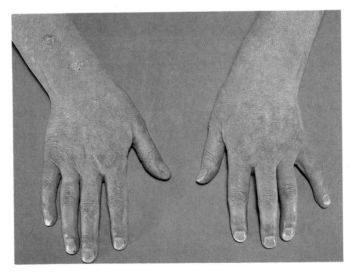

Fig. 6.10 A predominantly large joint pauciarticular arthritis with or without DIP involvement is also seen in Ps, as in this patient whose left wrist is involved as well as one ankle.

84

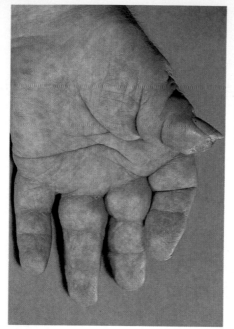

Fig. 6.11 Arthritis mutilans is the least common form of psoriatic arthritis. There is often gross osteolysis around the joints especially of the hands, producing the so-called telescopic finger. Function may be surprisingly well maintained.

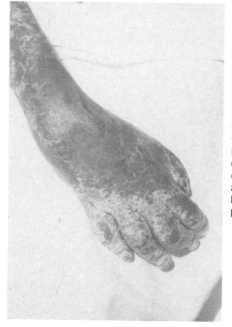

Fig. 6.12 Although skin disease and arthritis generally vary in activity independently of each other, occasional cases show a florid progression. In this young man, the entire skin surface was involved and the wrists, hands and knees were rapidly destroyed. Such cases need aggressive treatment but the prognosis is poor.

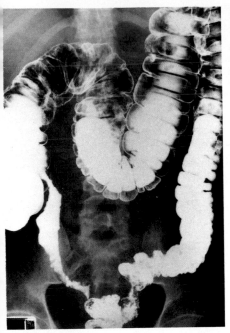

Fig. 6.13 A predominantly lower limb arthritis is seen in association with inflammatory bowel disease. This barium enema shows typical Crohn's disease with a narrowed terminal ileum (string sign) and a skip lesion in the sigmoid colon. The arthritis may move from one joint to another.

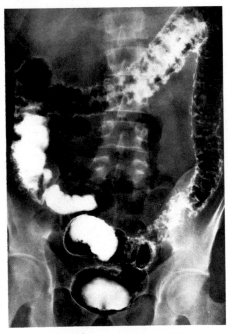

Fig. 6.14 Similar peripheral arthritis occurs with ulcerative colitis (UC), here typically involving the rectum and colon in continuity (i.e. no skip lesions). With both Crohn's disease and UC the peripheral arthritis and bowel lesions show parallel activity; a successful total colectomy in UC for example will usually abolish the arthritis.

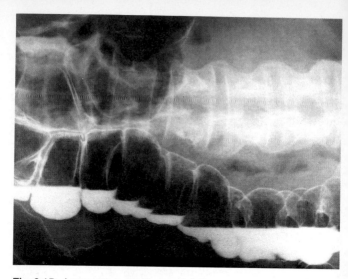

Fig. 6.15 A proportion of patients with inflammatory bowel disease also develop sacroiliitis and ankylosing spondylitis. This does not follow the activity of the bowel disease and tends to progress independently as can be seen from the ankylosed spine of this patient whose ulcerative colitis had been quiescent for many years.

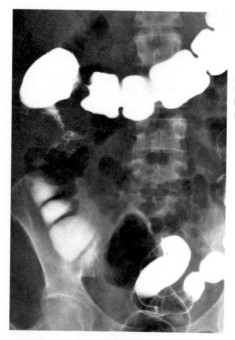

Fig. 6.16 Colonic carcinoma is a risk in patients with long-standing UC; here one is seen in the ascending colon. All UC patients should be kept under regular review.

Skin	Psoriasis Pustular psoriasis Keratoderma blennorrhagica	mainly palms and soles
Nails	Pitting, onycholysis or splitting	
Mucosal	Mouth ulcers – palate or tongue Balanitis	
Urethritis	Dysuria Clear or mucopurulent discharge Recent treatment for VD	
Bowels	History of bloody diarrhoea – Dysentery – Ulcerative colitis Colic and weight loss – Crohn's disease	
Eyes	Red, gritty eyes – Conjunctivitis Painful eyes, blurred vision – Uveitis	
Skeletal	Heel tenderness Back pain and stiffness, eased by exercise – Spondylitis	

Fig. 6.17 This check list may be of value in patients presenting with sero-negative asymmetrical arthritis. A careful examination and family history is rewarding as it may reveal the familial tendency of this diverse and fascinating group of conditions.

Aids for the disabled

The life of a disabled person can often be transformed by the provision of relatively simple aids and by advice on how to modify the house or its approaches to improve access and mobility, or how to adapt a car to facilitate driving despite a poor grip, painful shoulders or reduced cervical mobility. Many voluntary agencies offer such advice and in the UK it is also available through the Local Authority Social Services. All a doctor may need to do, therefore, is to point the disabled individual towards these services. Some knowledge of what is available is helpful both because it increases the likelihood of advice being offered and also because it improves the doctor's ability to talk about such matters with the patient, and thus improve his rapport. In this final section a small selection of the many possible aids is illustrated; further information is available in the many excellent pamphlets distributed through the voluntary agencies or from textbooks on rehabilitation. Rehabilitation is about adapting the environment to the patient just as much as about adapting the patient to his environment; often a little of both is required if his or her life is to be made as comfortable and independent as possible.

Expert help may be needed to provide additional hand rails for the stairs, to plumb-in a downstairs bathroom or to fit rails and raise flower beds in the garden. Adaptations at the place of work may require co-ordination between the doctor, the patient and the employer or a lighter job may have to be negotiated. Although social workers are often expert at organising such things, it is often the doctor who is the initiator; if he does not think of the various possibilities the patient may remain in ignorance, and much of the benefit of modern drug and surgical therapy diminished. Quality of life should be considered in its widest sense. Rheumatic conditions may sometimes be incurable and disabling but many patients continue to lead active, happy, fulfilling lives despite their disabilities.

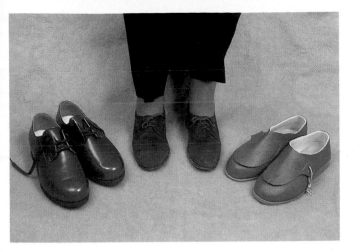

Fig. 7.1 Comfortable shoes which provide support and protection as well as adequate space for deformed feet are available in many different styles. Various types of temporary footwear (right) may be appropriate when surgery is being contemplated or if the patient requires surgical dressings for a while. Custom-made shoes with moulded insoles and soft, roomy uppers combine to improve mobility whilst reducing pain and risk of ulceration. They are expensive and require careful ordering.

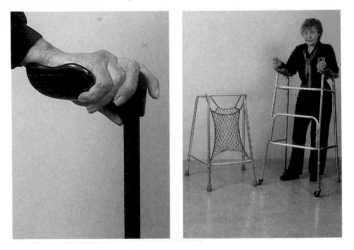

Fig. 7.2 A wide variety of walking aids is available. In addition to standard walking sticks, those with moulded handles may be more suited to patients with arthritic hands. Standard, elbow or gutter crutches are indicated in patients whose hand, wrist and elbow function is poor. For the more severely disabled, greater support and stability may be achieved by the use of tripod sticks or of various types of walking frame such as those illustrated.

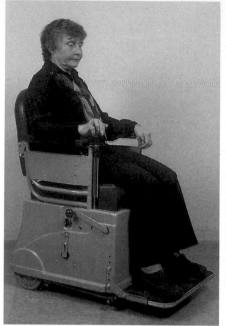

Fig. 7.3 Wheelchairs must be suited to the patient's needs – they may be self-propelling, propelled by a (fit) relative or friend, folding (if a car is available), or electric. Approaches to the home must be inspected and may need alteration with the addition of ramps. Interior doors may not be wide enough and a narrower chair may be provided if comfortable for the patient, or doors may have to be widened. Careful attention should be paid to providing correct seating and back rest.

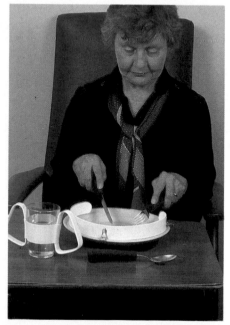

Fig. 7.4 Being fed is often felt to be a great indignity. Large-handled implements, a fork with a cutting edge, a non-slip mat to hold the plate and/or a removable plate rim all increase independence of feeding as do a variety of adapted mugs.

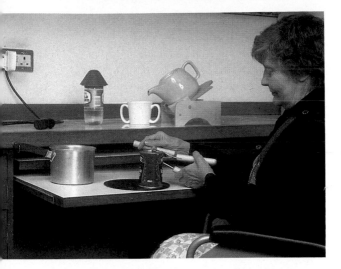

Fig. 7.5 For the disabled person to be able to prepare food, the provision of adapted surface heights with knee space, combined with a large number of labour-saving devices and handy gadgets may be necessary. The patient should be assessed at home by an occupational therapist both to ensure that the gadgets are being used properly and also to check that the arrangements are safe.

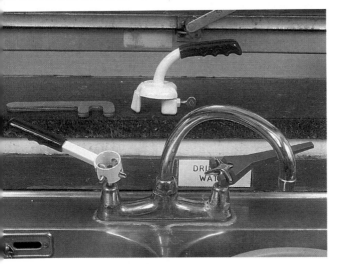

Fig. 7.6 Most designs of household tap require considerable grip combined with good wrist function. Lever adapters of the sort illustrated here are of great value in the kitchen and the bathroom. Hand rails, a bath or shower seat and a raised toilet seat are all important means of increasing the disabled person's privacy during personal toilet.

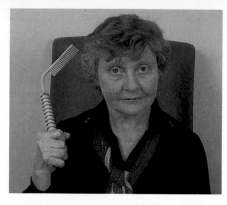

Fig. 7.7 When shoulder function is restricted, elongated handles are valuable and in situations where the patient is unable to bend easily, a 'helping hand' may be useful for picking up objects from the floor.

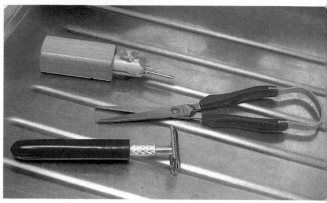

Fig. 7.8 With poor grip, everyday tools become difficult to use, but often simple solutions are available; a razor with a long non-slip handle, a pair of self-opening scissors, or a latch key with an enlarged grip are a few examples.

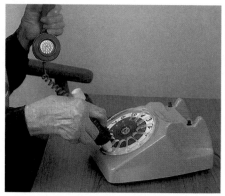

Fig. 7.9 Communication is particularly important to the disabled. A telephone may represent a major problem to someone with arthritic hands. This dialling stick or the provision of push-button dialling may greatly reduce the patient's feeling of isolation.

Index

Entries in **bold** refer to Fig. numbers